Earthing

If possible, read this book sitting with your bare feet
directly on the Earth—grass, gravel, dirt, sand, or concrete.

You will simultaneously experience what you are reading
about—how contact with the Earth restores your
body's natural electrical state.

The positive shift you feel is the start of a process in which
your body slowly becomes infused with the Earth's
omnipresent and ever-present healing energy.

This is Earthing, a remarkably simple, safe,
and natural act of reducing pain and stress.

*To the memory of Kay Wilson, who helped so, so much
in the early days of Earthing, and to all those many
other good people who saw that Earthing was
really something special and who gave me the needed
encouragement and support to carry on and bring this
knowledge to a world critically in need of it.*

—CLINTON OBER

*To my son, Step, who overcame near lethal electropollution
that ravaged six years of life and recovered with the help
of Earthing. You taught me so much about the tenacity
of the human spirit and how positive intention and
love can powerfully engage the healing process.
I am profoundly grateful for what you have taught me,
but infinitely more for the joy of still having you in my life.*

—STEPHEN SINATRA

*To Rosita, as always, and to the prospect of exploiting
our planet—for a change in a most magnificent way.*

—MARTIN ZUCKER

Foreword

By James L. Oschman, Ph.D.
Author of *Energy Medicine: The Scientific Basis* and
Energy Medicine in Therapeutics and Human Performance

This book unfolds an amazing story of discovery, a process that you, the reader, will soon experience for yourself as you read through the pages ahead.

It is a rare and humbling experience for a scientist to have the opportunity to explore new ground—and this story is all about ground—and participate in research that quickly infuses better health and more happiness into people's lives. It has been an exciting and challenging process for me. I was forced to ask questions that had never been asked before. The answers have ranged from fascinating to astounding, and they have shed light on some of the most important unsolved problems in physiology and medicine.

Among the many surprising revelations this book holds is an obvious, fundamental, and yet overlooked answer to the question of inflammation—recognized as the central health issue of our time—that surely will lay the foundation for many academic investigations and doctoral projects well into the future. I say that without equivocation, as an experienced academic cell biologist and biophysicist who has published dozens of articles in some of the world's leading scientific journals. The research in this book puts forward, and from a completely unexpected direction, a powerful reason for the proliferation of inflammation and, most importantly, what we can do about it.

As you read this book, you will quickly learn some profound and life-impacting facts you never knew before about our relationship with the planet we live on. You'll learn, for instance, how electrons play a central role in this relationship. The role of electrons in biology and health has long been my favorite subject. Of special importance in my explorations of the electronic aspects of life was an association during the 1980s with the leading research group studying this subject, consisting of Nobel Laureate Albert Szent-Györgyi and colleagues from around the world at the Marine Biological Laboratory in Woods Hole, Massachusetts. A number of these great inquiring minds were electronic engineers and materials scientists recruited to study a field he created and named *electronic biology*. Dr. Szent-Györgyi was considered one of the leading scientists of the twentieth century, and his research and writings have been a continuing source of inspiration and insight. I have published a series of articles and two books on the ways electrons can move about within the human body and the ways various therapeutic methods influence electron motions. The research summarized in this book adds a whole new dimension to our understandings of electronic biology.

This book traces the discoveries of Clinton Ober, a pioneer in the cable TV industry, who uncovered the health benefits of Earthing—his term for connecting ourselves to the surface of our planet by sitting, standing, or walking barefoot on the Earth or by sleeping on special conductive sheets and pads connected to a simple metal rod stuck in the ground outside a bedroom window. Clint invented these sleep systems and a number of other devices that help us to restore a vital but previously overlooked connection with Mother Earth.

Many people describe a sense of well-being when they walk barefoot on the Earth. The stories and the research in the book reveal the background, dynamics, and implications of this feel-good sensation, a real experience indicative of something profoundly important that most of us have been missing in our lives. This missing link is so profound in fact that it seems to do away with or dramatically improve so many health challenges common in this day and age: insomnia, the chronic pain of multiple diseases and injuries, exhaustion, stress, anxiety, and premature aging. I was quickly and enthusiastically drawn into this research when I saw how many people experienced a wide variety of health benefits from simply connecting their bodies to the Earth. Especially impressive has been the experience my physician friend and colleague, Jeff Spencer, D.C., has had during the spectacular series of victories of the American cycling teams in the Tour de France. You'll read about Jeff's remarkable story later in the book. These observations were augmented with my personal observations of many friends who benefited from the application of Earthing systems in their lives. When my massage therapist began using Earthing with her clients she achieved so many successes that physicians in the area began sending her their most difficult cases to treat. My own challenge was to determine precisely how Earthing produces such benefits and to find a way of explaining this accurately in the language of science.

Our research on Earthing has uncovered what is perhaps the most simple and natural remedy against proliferating, painful, and often deadly conditions, including the diseases of aging, created by various kinds of inflammation. As you will read further on, our hypothesis for how this remedy works is unlike any you have ever heard. In all its ramifications, we think it represents a new healing paradigm.

In short, Earthing restores and maintains the human body's most natural electrical state, which in turn promotes optimum health and functionality in daily life. The primordial natural energy emanating from the Earth is the ultimate anti-inflammatory and the ultimate anti-aging medicine.

For more than a decade, Clint Ober has tirelessly pursued a one-man mission to awaken a skeptical world to a simple and forgotten fact: that the Earth beneath our feet contains great healing energy and that connecting ourselves to this energy is immediately beneficial as well as intuitively and remarkably simple.

As with any new discovery, Clint had to endure skepticism and derision from "experts," some of whom regarded him as crazy. But he persisted and has now gathered significant scientific evidence for his out-of-the-box idea. Moreover, thousands of people who have applied the concept of Earthing in their lives feel, look, and sleep better, and they have less pain.

As we explored absolutely new avenues of research in order to validate the concept of Earthing and determine how it affects the human body, Clint turned out to be a rock solid and dedicated guide to those of us with Ph.D.s after our names. Clint often refers to his lack of education as a scientist, but what he has accomplished shows that determined and inspired individuals can accomplish an enormous amount by teaching themselves what they need to know. I have been continually astonished by Clint's precise and accurate insights that go beyond the conclusions a logical scientific mind would usually develop. I feel that I have been privileged to work with a genuine discoverer and pioneer whose interest in helping others exceeds any personal interest by far.

Steve Sinatra, a Connecticut cardiologist who specializes in integrative medicine and has an interest in electromedicine, met Clint in 2001 and saw great promise for Earthing in his own field of cardiology, as well as medicine in general. Steve encouraged Clint to stick with it and pursue research, particularly the connection with inflammation, which had been recently found to be the probable cause of heart disease.

Persist he did. Eventually, Clint found open-minded experts in the fields of medicine, physiology, and biophysics, and inspired a series of research projects showing that the surface of the Earth is like one gigantic anti-inflammatory, sleep booster, and energizer—all wrapped up in one.

Now, Clint, Steve, and veteran health writer Martin Zucker have teamed up to present the exciting story of Earthing and how it can help all of us Earthlings.

To break new ground means to do something different from anything done before. If ever the term *groundbreaking* applies to a book, it certainly does here, literally and figuratively. This book is about the ground beneath our feet, and the revelation of a vital electrical continuum between the Earth and the living organisms that dwell upon it.

Walk, stand, and sit barefoot on the ground for a half hour or so. If you have PMS or arthritic pain or a backache or indigestion or jet lag or are just feeling fatigued, go outside (weather permitting, of course) with your bare feet placed directly on the Earth.

At the end of that time you will feel better. And as you feel better, a lightbulb will go off in your head. You will realize that although you live on the surface of the Earth your lifestyle has separated you from the limitless healing energy that, unknown to you, the surface beneath your feet holds. It's there, and always there, and yours for the taking.

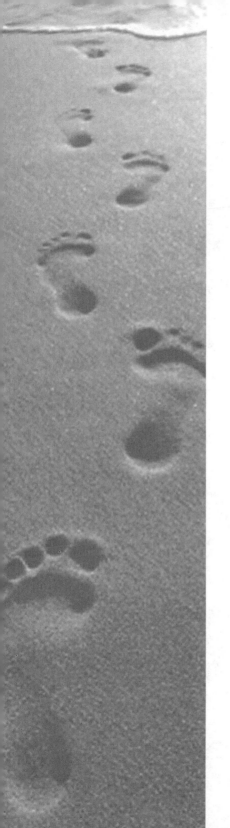

PART ONE

Why We Are Unhealthy— The Missing Link

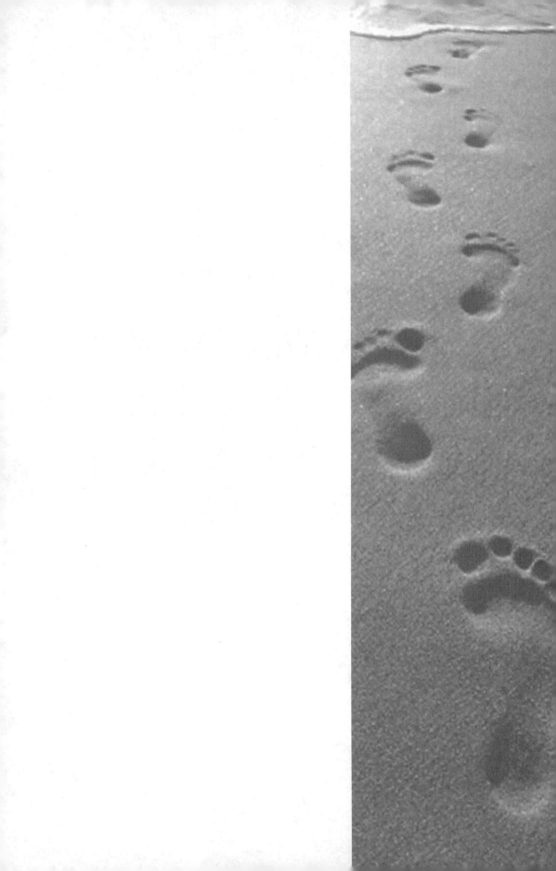

CHAPTER 1

Electrical You and Your Electrical Planet

Have you ever noticed a subtle tingling or sensation of warmth rising up from your feet during a barefoot stroll on a sandy beach or grassy field glistening with the morning dew?

Did you feel revitalized at the end of your walk?

If you did, you experienced the Earth energizing your body.

The fact is that we live on a planet alive with natural energies. Its surface teems with subtly pulsating frequencies, a phenomenon unknown to most people. Who regards the sand, grass, sidewalk, or dirt beneath their feet as an energy field?

But that indeed is what the ground is and always has been.

Put another way, your planet is a six sextillion (that's six followed by twenty-one zeroes) metric ton battery that is continually being replenished by solar radiation, lightning, and heat from its deep-down molten core. And just like a battery in a car that keeps the motor running and the wheels turning, so, too, do the rhythmic pulsations of natural energy flowing through and emanating from the surface of the Earth keep the biological machinery of global life running in rhythm and balance—for everything that lives on the land or in the sea.

People.

Animals.

Fish.

Plants.

Trees.

Bugs.

Bacteria.

Viruses.

Throughout history, humans have strolled, sat, stood, and slept on the ground—the skin of their bodies touching the skin of the Earth—oblivious to the fact that such simple contact transfers a natural electrical signal to the body.

Only recently has the knowledge and significance of this connection been explored and explained by scientific experts in geophysics, biophysics, electrical engineering, electrophysiology, and medicine. From them, we are learning that the Earth's electrical energy maintains the order of our own bodily frequencies just as a conductor controls the coherence and cadence of an orchestra. We all live and function electrically on an electrical planet. We are each of us a collection of dynamic electrical circuits. In the living matrix of our complex bodies, trillions of cells constantly transmit and receive energy in the course of their programmed biochemical reactions. Think of them as microscopic electronic machines. The movement of nutrients and water into the cells is regulated by electric fields, and each type of cell has a frequency range in which it operates. Your heart, brain, nervous system, muscles, and immune system are prime examples of electrical subsystems operating within your "bioelectrical" body. The fact is, all of your movements, behaviors, and actions are energized by electricity.

OUR LOST ELECTRICAL ROOTS

Most people, even in this scientific age, are totally unaware of their bioelectrical nature. Practically no one has the slightest notion of an electrical or energetic connection between his or her body and the Earth. Nobody learns about it in school. So nobody knows that we have largely become disconnected and separated from the Earth. In developed societies, in particular, we have essentially lost our electrical roots. Our bare feet, with their rich network of nerve endings, rarely touch the ground. We wear insulating synthetic-soled shoes. We sleep on elevated beds made from insulating material. Most of us in the modern, industrialized world live disconnected from the Earth's surface. Although it is not something you probably have ever thought about, you may be suffering needlessly because of this disconnect. And you may be suffering severely, and in more ways than you could ever imagine.

As an analogy, think of a lightbulb with a loose connection. The bulb flickers, shines weakly, or doesn't light up at all. Many people go through life with flickering or weak health.

We believe this book is the first ever written about Mother Earth's natural "vibes" and how they keep us healthy and heal us—if we connect to the source. Disconnected, the body seems vulnerable and prone to dysfunction, inflammation-related disease, and accelerated aging—a startling theory just beginning to gather scientific momentum.

This is the subject of our book.

The natural frequencies of the Earth that we speak of are waves of energy caused by the motions of subatomic particles called free electrons. Nobody has ever seen an electron, but you can think of them in the setting of a beehive. The bees, buzzing around the hive, are like electrons that move around the atomic nucleus in a "cloud" of energy. Another analogy used over the years is that of planets revolving around the sun. The nucleus contains protons, with a positive charge, and neutrons, that have, as their name implies, no charge. Electrons have a negative charge.

ELECTRICALLY CONDUCTIVE YOU

To understand the primordial relationship between bioelectrical you and your electrical planet, consider for a brief moment three types of materials used in electricity: conductors, insulators, and semiconductors. An example of a conductor is the metallic copper wiring in the walls of your house or in the electrical cord that you plug into an outlet from an appliance. The outer waves of electrons in conductors—corresponding in a simplistic way to the outermost bees buzzing around the beehive or to the distant planets orbiting around the sun—are so loosely bound that they easily move in the space between the atoms. They form a kind of gas around atoms and flow freely throughout the solid conductive material. That is why they are called free electrons. Think of them as free spirits, so to speak, not bound in a relationship with any atom composing the solid material.

In insulating materials, electrons are held in a tight grip by their atoms. There are no free electrons and consequently no current can flow through these materials. Examples of insulating materials include plastic, rubber,

glass, and wood. You can now see why most of the time you are separated from the Earth. Your shoes' soles are made of plastic or rubber, and
your house is made mainly of wood. Semiconductors are in between, sometimes conducting, sometimes not. Their electrical conductance is not as
good as a conductor but not as bad as an insulator. Semiconductors are
the backbone of modern electronic equipment because their conductance
can be controlled by the application of an electric field.

Just like the Earth, your body is mostly water and minerals, and both
are excellent conductors of electrons. The free electrons pulsating perpetually on the surface of the conductive Earth, fed by natural phenomenon—solar radiation, thousands of lightning strikes per minute, and
energy generated from the inner core of the planet—are easily transferred
up, into, and throughout your body as long as there is *direct skin contact*
with the ground.

Homo erectus, back a hundred thousand generations or so, didn't know
a thing about any of this. Neither did the hunter-gatherers who followed
in the human timeline. Neither did the cultivator civilizations working
the land about four hundred generations ago. And neither did the more
recent Industrial Age incarnations. Even in today's electronic and wireless
age, few know about the Earth's brimming reservoir of energetic free
electrons.

Scientists back in the late 1800s first measured the Earth's subtle ground
currents at different places around the world, using words such as "tran-
quil" and "quiet" to describe them. Present-day science refers to them as
"telluric currents" and recognizes them as part of a larger system—called
the "global electrical circuit"—involving clouds and the entire atmosphere.
Geophysicists believe that this bank of almost limitless energy is continuously replenished with free electrons via an average of 5,000 lightning
strikes per minute occurring perpetually around the planet. Without getting technical, the electrical potential present on the Earth's surface rises
and falls according to the position of the sun. The intensity is more positive and energetic during the day, in support of your daily activities from
wake up to shut down, and less positive and energetic during nighttime
hours, promoting zzzzzzs. This daily high and low pattern sets in motion
and orchestrates internal body mechanisms that regulate sleep-wake cycles,
hormone production, and maintenance of health.

PAST CONNECTIONS

The basic phenomena of electricity were known since antiquity, but electricity was only harnessed for industrial and residential use about 120 years ago or so. The electron itself was discovered only in 1897, so virtually throughout the human timeline nobody knew anything about electrons. But there was plenty of knowledge over the eons of time that the ground held special healing energy and was a basic aspect of connectedness to Nature. The Earth was sacred. This knowledge, passed down over the generations, has survived in one form or another around the globe. Civilizations everywhere recognized and tuned in to the cycles of Nature for survival and health. They were aware of fundamental rhythms that regulate, for instance, sleep-wake cycles and maintenance of health, and they knew that we functioned in coordination with the Earth's cycles and rhythms. Awareness existed of connectivity among the principles of Earth, life, and health, but expressed in the language of the day.

Qi (pronounced *chee*) is a central principle in the long history of Chinese knowledge and is regarded as the energy or natural force that fills the universe. From India's Vedic past comes an equivalent term, *prana*, meaning "vital force."

In the Chinese tradition, Heaven Qi is made up of the forces that heavenly bodies exert on the Earth, such as sunshine, moonlight, and the moon's effect on the tides. Earth Qi, influenced and controlled by Heaven Qi, is made up of lines and patterns of energy, as well as the Earth's magnetic field and the heat concealed underground. And within the Earth Qi, individuals, animals, and plants have their own Qi field. All natural things, in this concept, grow and are influenced by the natural cycles of Heaven Qi and Earth Qi.

Earth Qi is absorbed, without thinking about it, when we walk barefoot, which may explain why it's so relaxing to walk without shoes and why exercises geared toward strengthening the body and relaxing the mind (yoga, tai chi, and qigong, for instance) are often practiced without footwear. A central focus in Chinese practices involves "growing a root" and has to do with opening up communication between the bottom of the feet and the Earth. This process occurs through the "yong quan point," also known in acupuncture as the "kidney 1 point."

The ancient Greeks surely knew something about this concept. Hercules, one of the greatest heroes of Greek mythology, fought and defeated the giant Antaeus, who was renowned as a great wrestler. As the story goes, Antaeus was invincible as long as his feet remained in contact with the Earth, from where he drew his strength. He had never been defeated. Hercules, knowing Antaeus' secret, lifts the giant off the ground and strangles him to death.

Native Americans certainly honored the connection to the Earth. The late Ota Kte (Luther Standing Bear), a writer, educator, and tribal leader from the Lakota Sioux tradition, summed it up this way: "The old people came literally to love the soil. They sat on the ground with the feeling of being close to a mothering power. It was good for the skin to touch the Earth, and the old people liked to remove their moccasins and walk with their bare feet on the sacred Earth. The soil was soothing, strengthening, cleansing, and healing."

CONNECT TO THE EARTH AND HEAL

This book will show you just how soothing, strengthening, and healing the Earth is. It will totally change the way you regard the ground under your feet and your relationship to the planet you live on.

For most people, reconnecting with Mother Earth usually means camping, hiking, gardening, going to the beach, or pursuing some other activity that returns us—in body and soul—to the bosom of Nature. The reconnection we talk about in this book is something different. By reconnection we mean taking off your shoes and socks and sitting, standing, or walking barefoot on the ground, something that is absolutely free and available (of course, where safe and comfortable). The reconnection can also involve the use of conductive bed sheets or floor pads linked by wire to a ground rod outside your house or office, or plugged into a wall outlet with a modern Earth ground system.

Either way, we call this reconnection process "Earthing" or "grounding," terms we will use interchangeably. They simply mean you are connected to Mother Earth. What you are doing is akin to what is well known in the electrical world as grounding, the common practice of connecting equipment and appliances to the Earth to protect against shocks, shorts, and interference. Applied to people, Earthing naturally protects the body's delicate bioelectrical circuitry against static electrical charges and interference. Most importantly, it facilitates the reception of free electrons and the stabilizing electrical signals and energy of the Earth. Earthing remedies an electrical instability and electron deficiency you never knew you had. It refills and recharges your body with something you never knew you were missing . . . or needed.

Exposure to sunlight produces vitamin D in the body. It's needed for health. Exposure to the ground provides an electrical "nutrient" in the form of electrons. Think of these electrons as vitamin G—G for ground. Just like vitamin D, you need vitamin G for your health as well.

As you will read in this book, the results of Earthing often translate into a significant improvement—even total transformations—in health and vitality. One patient, a thirty-six-year-old woman with advanced multiple sclerosis (MS), was so happy about her improvement after Earthing that she once ran out of her house, stood in the middle of the street, and screamed to all her neighbors to get grounded. She said she wanted to start the "barefoot revolution" and teach everyone how to get well. She had tried Earthing out of desperation—something someone had told her about —after a doctor advised her to purchase an adjustable bed, a large screen television, and to make herself as comfortable as possible. MS doesn't get better, the doctor told her. In her case it did, and dramatically so.

Another woman spent over five years with debilitating pain, inflammation, fatigue, and sleep problems after a serious car accident. Despite a long career in the health care industry, she found herself locked in an exhausting struggle to regain her health. She went from one practitioner and treatment to another. "Like Humpty Dumpty in the nursery rhyme," she said, "all of the king's horses and all the king's men could not put me back together again." Unable to work, she found herself instinctively drawn to lying in the grass or walking barefoot on the beach. In 1999, a friend gave her a conductive bed pad. She slept on it nightly, and within months her pain, fatigue, and sleep problems vanished.

"After years of pills and failed costly treatments, all I did was lay down on my bed and sleep!" she said. "I believe our bodies have the ability to recover from almost any condition if we relieve imbalances caused by stress. To do this, we must provide our bodies with essential natural elements,

Earthing at a Glance

What is Earthing?

Earthing involves coupling your body to the Earth's eternal and gentle surface energies. It means walking barefoot outside and/or sitting, working or sleeping inside while connected to a conductive device that delivers the natural healing energy of the Earth into your body. For more than ten years, thousands of people around the world—men, women, children, and athletes—have incorporated Earthing into their daily routines. The results have been documented and they are extraordinary.

What isn't Earthing?

You are not in any sense being electrocuted. Earthing is among the most natural and safest things you can do.

What happens?

Your body becomes suffused with negative-charged free electrons abundantly present on the surface of the Earth. Your body immediately equalizes to the same electric energy level, or potential, as the Earth.

What do you feel?

Sometimes, a warm, tingling sensation and often feelings of ease and well-being.

Will you feel better?

Usually, yes, and often rapidly. The degree of improvement varies from person to person. The important thing is to make Earthing a long-term addition to your daily routine, and to do it as much as possible so as to gain maximum benefits. When Earthing is stopped, symptoms tend to slowly return.

What does Earthing do?

Observations and research indicate the following benefits from Earthing; we expect many more to emerge with ongoing studies. Earthing:

- Defuses the cause of inflammation, and improves or eliminates the symptoms of many inflammation-related disorders.

- Reduces or eliminates chronic pain.

- Improves sleep in most cases.

- Increases energy.

- Lowers stress and promotes calmness in the body by cooling down the nervous system and stress hormones.

- Normalizes the body's biological rhythms.

- Thins blood and improves blood pressure and flow.

- Relieves muscle tension and headaches.

- Lessens hormonal and menstrual symptoms.

- Dramatically speeds healing and helps prevent bedsores.

- Reduces or eliminates jet lag.

- Protects the body against potentially health-disturbing environmental electromagnetic fields (EMFs).

- Accelerates recovery from intense athletic activity.

including clean air, proper nutrition and pure water, and the missing link, our connection to the natural electrical rhythms of the Earth."

Even athletes, who operate at the most intense levels of physical human performance, have learned to ground and plug in to the natural energy of the Earth. From a group perspective, perhaps the most dramatic test of Earthing's effectiveness in recent years was demonstrated by victorious American-sponsored cycling teams at the Tour de France. The extreme physical and mental stress in this grueling race often causes sickness, tendonitis, and poor sleep among competitors. They tend to experience slow wound healing from accidents. In the 2003 to 2005 races, and again in 2007, team cyclists were grounded after their daily competition. They reported better sleep, significantly less illness, practically no tendonitis, dramatic recovery from the day's racing, and faster healing of injuries. The practice has now been found to be so beneficial that many top athletes— including swimmers, NFL football players, triathletes, and motorcycle racers—routinely Earth themselves.

Earthing is simple, basic, and powerful. We regard it as a genuine miss-ing link in the health equation, something with astounding potential to do much good for humanity. Connecting to the Earth—either by being barefooted outside or in contact with a grounded device inside—doesn't cure you of any disease or condition. What it does is to reunite you with the natural electrical signals from the Earth that govern all organisms dwelling upon it. It restores your body's natural internal electrical stabil-ity and rhythms, which in turn promote normal functioning of body sys-tems, including the cardiovascular, respiratory, digestive, and immune systems. It remedies an electron deficiency to reduce inflammation—the common cause of disease. It shifts the nervous system from a stress-dominated mode to one of calmness and you sleep better. By reconnect-ing, you enable your body to return to its normal electrical state, better able to self-regulate and self-heal.

In 1863, the eminent biologist T. H. Huxley stated that "the question of all questions for humanity, the problem which lies behind all others and is more interesting than any of them, is that of the determination of our place in nature and our relation to the cosmos." The content of this book explores that question from the simple perspective that your place in nature, in your immediate cosmos, requires you to be directly and rou-tinely connected to the Earth under your feet.

In the pages ahead, we will explore the health implications of mankind's disconnect and present the unusual story about how the disconnect and the reconnect were discovered. You will read accounts of amazing healing from doctors and people from all walks of life. Most importantly, you will learn how easy it is to reconnect, to get Earthed, and to feel better.

CHAPTER 2

The Disconnect Syndrome

Illnesses do not come upon us out of the blue.
They are developed from small daily sins against Nature.
When enough sins have accumulated, illnesses will suddenly appear.
—HIPPOCRATES

The father of medicine clearly knew what he was talking about 2,500 years ago when he saw his Greek countrymen committing all kinds of sins against Nature. Imagine what he would think today just by looking at the most supposedly advanced country in the world. U.S. medical expenses, public and private, account for more than 17 percent of the gross national product and are projected to grow at a rate of 6 percent a year. By 2018, our medical bill will represent 20 percent of the country's earnings!

Ouch. That implies a lot of sickness and an inability of the medical system to prevent disease in the first place. Hippocrates would likely say there's a mighty amount of sinning going on.

In today's scientific age, an intense debate reverberates among researchers over what's to blame for the alarming increase in immune- and inflammation-related diseases.

In March 2008, an article by Rob Stein of the *Washington Post* brought attention to one of the primary issues responsible for the health meltdown: the decline of the human immune system. His article was entitled "Is Modern Life Ravaging Our Immune Systems?"

"First, asthma cases shot up, along with hay fever and other common allergic reactions, such as eczema," Mr. Stein wrote. "Then pediatricians started seeing more children with food allergies. Now experts are increasingly convinced that a suspected jump in lupus, multiple sclerosis, and other afflictions caused by misfiring immune systems is real.

"Although the data are stronger for some diseases than others, and part of the increase may reflect better diagnoses, experts estimate that many allergies and immune-system diseases have doubled, tripled, or even quadrupled in the past few decades, depending on the ailment and the country. Some studies now indicate that more than half of the U.S. population has at least one allergy."

Researchers are leveling blame at modern living because the increases have shown up first largely in highly developed nations in Europe, North America, and elsewhere, and they are on the rise in other countries as they become more developed.

"It's striking," one British researcher said.

"Disturbing," said one French researcher, referring to the increase of autoimmune disorders, the difficult to treat and often disabling conditions stemming from a dysfunctional immune system that attacks the body's own cells, tissues, and organs. Common autoimmune diseases include lupus, rheumatoid arthritis, multiple sclerosis, and type 1 diabetes. The cause remains unknown, and the reasons for the increase are poorly understood. Collectively, they are among the most prevalent diseases in the United States, afflicting between 15 and 24 million people, about 75 percent of them women.

THE RISE OF INFLAMMATION

All these conditions—as well as the major disease killers like cardiovascular disease, type 2 diabetes, and cancer—are linked to chronic inflammation, a subject that has taken over center court in medical research during the last few years. As *Time* magazine reported in a 2004 cover article, "Hardly a week goes by without the publication of yet another study uncovering a new way that chronic inflammation does harm to the body." It torches the sensitive linings of the arteries that feed the heart and brain, leading to heart attacks and stroke. It chews up nerve cells in the brain and may contribute to the development of dementia and Alzheimer's disease. It can promote the proliferation of abnormal cells and facilitate their conversion into cancer. "In other words," the magazine said, "chronic inflammation may be the engine that drives many of the most feared illnesses of middle and old age."

The rise of inflammation in medical awareness has spawned a new term: "inflamm-aging." Italian researchers coined it in 2006 to describe a progressive inflammatory status and a loss of stress-coping ability as two major characteristics of the aging process.

Inflammation is now believed to be the underlying cause of more than eighty chronic illnesses, and more than half of Americans suffer currently from one or more of them. Each year, millions die from these conditions. The most common chronic diseases cost the U.S. economy alone more than $1 trillion annually—and that figure threatens to reach $6 trillion by the middle of the century.

"Inflammation may turn out to be the elusive Holy Grail of medicine— the single phenomenon that holds the key to sickness and health," wrote William Meggs, M.D., Ph.D., of East Carolina University in his book *The Inflammation Cure: How to Combat the Hidden Factor Behind Heart Disease, Arthritis, Asthma, Diabetes & Other Diseases* (McGraw-Hill, 2003).

THE MISSING LINK

What is clear in all this is that the immune system is being overwhelmed. The usual suspects in the scientific debate include genetics, poor diet, air pollution, obesity, physical inactivity, and even living in sterile homes. What has become evident to us is that researchers have overlooked another factor, something right under their noses, or to be more anatomically specific, right under their feet. In this book, we propose to add something new to the list of offenders: the lost connection to our planet's natural flow of surface electrical energy and the electron deficiency in our bodies this creates. Our investigations strongly suggest that the incidence of soaring chronic diseases during our lifetimes has occurred during a period in which more and more people have become increasingly disconnected from the Earth.

Is this disconnect and deficiency a missing link, an overlooked reason why sickness statistics rise ever higher? Is it perhaps the biggest cause of all? If inflammation is the Holy Grail of medicine, is connection to the Earth the Holy Grail of inflammation?

The answer to the first question is a resounding *yes.*

We don't presume to know yet the answer to the second and third questions. That will take years of investigation, but the initial research, along with many real life observations and experiences, provides intriguing evidence. This book is filled with that evidence. We believe that the information collected on the pages ahead packs the potential to reverse an alarming trend of failing health. We also think it can inspire entire new health standards and businesses based on reconnecting large segments of disconnected populations. We are sure that this information, if widely applied, can help any and all efforts to ease the health care burden shouldered by individuals, employers, and governments alike—literally from the ground up.

The evidence we have gathered strongly suggests that your health status stands to benefit in multiple ways when you reconnect, even if you are chronically and seriously sick and the medical system has little to offer you.

The human immune system evolved over millions of years. During this great span of time, of course, we lived mostly in barefoot contact with the Earth. We were naturally Earthed. Yet scientists haven't noticed that modern living involves a disconnect with Earth's stabilizing electrical energy and a loss of the body's natural grounded state, and that *this* loss may set up the immune system for malfunction.

Did the immune system—and the nervous system and other systems in the body—stop functioning properly when we began wearing shoes with insulating soles and living inside houses that insulate us from the natural frequencies of the environment?

Disconnecting Experimentally

What happens to the human body when it is separated from the subtle evolutionary signals from the Earth was dramatically shown by experiments in Germany at the world-famous Max Planck Institute during the 1960s and 1970s. Researchers intentionally isolated volunteers for months at a time in underground rooms electrically shielded from the rhythms in the Earth's electric field. Patterns of body temperature, sleep, urinary excretion, and other physiological activities were carefully monitored. All the participants developed a variety of abnormal or chaotic patterns, sort of like a head-to-toe arrhythmia. They experienced disturbed sleep and waking patterns, out-of-sync hormonal production, and overall a disruption in basic body regulation.

When electric rhythms comparable to those measured at the Earth's surface were pulsed into the metal shielding around the underground chambers, there was a dramatic restoration of normal physiological patterns.

These studies, involving hundreds of participants over many years, clearly documented the significance of the Earth's electrical rhythms for normal biological function. Normal rhythms in the body establish a stable reference point for repair, recovery, and rejuvenation—in short, for full health.

Clearly, the biological chaos induced in the experiments would lead in time to ill health. The conclusion is that the biological clock of the body needs to be continually calibrated by the pulse of the Earth that governs the circadian rhythms of all life on the planet.

Experiments like these, under controlled conditions, provide dramatic evidence. Yet we don't live underground. We live above the ground but not really on the ground—and that's the problem. We're disconnected. You can perhaps look at yourself and many people around you and get an idea of the consequences of this disconnect. There's a lot of sickness. Just read the health—rather, disease—statistics and you will see more evidence that in large or small part indicates a disconnect syndrome.

How are we disconnected even though we obviously live on the planet?

The Shoe Problem

Look at what you put on your feet on a daily basis. Most of you wear one form or another of footwear that evolved from simple foot coverings designed to protect against chilly and challenging ground conditions. You are likely wearing something much more elaborate, a statement reflecting your culture, fashion, behavior, and, in many cases, even identification with a tennis or basketball superstar. You habitually wear shoes even when they do not serve any practical purpose.

The late Dr. William Rossi, a Massachusetts podiatrist, footwear industry historian, prolific author, and keen observer, wrote many disturbing commentaries on what shoes do to our feet. He strongly believed that footwear is an integral part of foot care and often complained that shoe people didn't understand feet and foot-care people didn't understand shoes.

A "natural gait is biomechanically impossible for any shoe-wearing person," he wrote in a 1999 article in *Podiatry Management.* "It took four million years to develop our unique human foot and our consequent distinctive form of gait, a remarkable feat of bioengineering. Yet, in only a few thousand years, and with one carelessly designed instrument, our shoes, we have warped the pure anatomical form of human gait, obstructing its engineering efficiency, afflicting it with strains and stresses and denying it its natural grace of form and ease of movement head to foot."

Mechanical issues aside, Dr. Rossi was uncommonly attuned to the potential health risks caused by the separation of the Earth and the body created by modern shoes with soles made of insulating material.

"The sole (or plantar surface) of the foot is richly covered with some 1,300 nerve endings per square inch," he wrote in a 1997 article in *Footwear News.* "That's more than found on any other part of the body of comparable size. Why are so many nerve endings concentrated there? To keep us 'in touch' with the Earth. The real physical world around us. It's called 'sensory response.' The foot is the vital link between the person and the Earth. The paws of all animals are equally rich in nerve endings. The Earth is covered with an electromagnetic layer. It's this that creates the sensory response in our feet and [in] the paws of animals. Try walking barefoot on the ground for a couple of minutes. Every living thing, including human beings, draws energy from this field through its feet, paws, or roots."

Dr. Rossi referred to the foot "as a kind of radar-sonic base" providing a "little-known but vital function" that serves to "extract" energy from the Earth, similar to a plant root extracting moisture from the ground for nourishment. Such "ground-to-foot vibrations may thus be an important energizing power helping to serve the body's life forces," he suggested.

How right he was, even though he was mistaken in thinking that the source of this energy being drawn up into the body was magnetic. It is now well established that the energy residing on the surface of the Earth is primarily electrical. The central theme of our book is that we draw electrical energy through our feet in the form of free electrons fluctuating at many frequencies. These frequencies reset our biological clock and provide the body with electrical energy. The electrons themselves flow into the body, equalizing and maintaining it at the electrical potential of the Earth. Just like standard electronic equipment that needs a stable ground to function well, so, too, the body needs stable grounding to also function well.

Dr. Rossi bemoaned the fact that modern shoe soles have separated us from the energy and feeling of the ground, which is so important to the foot's sensory response. He wrote: "The bottoms of our footwear are virtually 'deadened.' A cross section of a shoe reveals several layers: outsole, midsole, insole filler material, footbed, cushioning, sockliner. An almost total blockout of sensory response."

Dr. Rossi's lament describes in a few words the post-World War II overhaul of shoe making. New materials entered the manufacturing scene: rubber, plastic, and petrochemical compounds. They have slowly squeezed out leather as the historical source of shoe soles. Nowadays, even makers of fancy men's dress shoes are increasingly switching to rubber, plastic, and other non-conductive material, just as casual and work shoes before them. Leather (processed from hides), a conductive material when moist, has been the traditional source of shoes and sandals. The original lightweight, softsole, heel-less and simple moccasin—a piece of crudely tanned leather that envelops the foot and is fastened on with rawhide thongs—is possibly the closest we have ever come to an "ideal" shoe. It dates back more than 14,000 years.

In his writings, Dr. Rossi also noted another intriguing connection between the foot and the ground—an erotic connection. The human foot, he wrote, is "rich with vibratory and electromagnetic powers linked to Earth contact—which is one reason for its age-old association with human fertility and the reproductive system."

The foot, he pointed out in his 1989 book, *The Sex Life of the Foot and Shoe* (Wentworth edition), is a primary sense organ lavishly equipped with "sexual nerves" and "every moment of standing or walking involves sensory contact with the ground." Erotic sensations "can be aroused by the

The "World's Most Dangerous Invention"

David Wolfe, an author, speaker, and outspoken authority on health and lifestyle, deems "the common shoe" as perhaps the "world's most dangerous invention." After fifteen years of nutritional and lifestyle research, he incriminates the shoe as one of the "most destructive culprits of inflammation and autoimmune diseases" in our lives because it separates us from the healing energy of the Earth.

"Put a shoe on," he says, "and it's gone."

touch of Earth, grass, wind, air, sun, sand, water. Such a sensation is experienced when you remove your shoes and stockings on a warm day and walk barefoot on the grass or sand, or dip your feet into a cool pool. The exhilaration is strongly sensual."

Beds and Beyond

For the most part, the modern structures we live and do business in—our homes and workplaces—are also non-conductive and separate us from the Earth's healing electrons. Think about where you spend most of your day: in an apartment, house, or office elevated off the ground, with a layer of wood, synthetic carpeting, or vinyl covering the floor. Unless you live on a dirt, cement, marble, or stone floor, it is unlikely that you are receiving any good vibes from below. We'll discuss later how living and working in multi-story edifices may create a risk to health.

Like shoes and houses, beds, too, have evolved. They further separate most of us nowadays from the Earth for the third of the time we spend sleeping. We sleep (or toss and turn, as is the case for the masses of insomniacs) on nice and comfy padded elevated beds, in elevated houses, avoiding creeping and crawling things in the night.

The first record of raised beds is associated with the Egyptian pharaohs and their wealthy friends, thanks to the innovations of local Bronze Age craftsmen (3,000–1,000 BC). Although the fashion and the bedding has changed in the centuries since, the simple concept of sleeping on a platform resting on four legs hasn't changed much.

Before the Egyptians, however, humans apparently snuggled up for the night on the ground and, of course, where accessible, in nice, dry caves. Believe it or not, in this modern age there are still cave dwellers around, most notably 40 million or so in mountainous north-central China. They live surrounded by the Earth, and the Earth's energy, and as we have heard, even with cable TV.

Anthropologists tell us they discovered evidence of grass-lined beds dating back over nine thousand years in southwest Texas. Pits were created in the soft sediment with grass piled in for some crude level of comfort. Whether straw, grass, or sleeping skins, these natural materials, when combined with perspiration from the body, have accommodated electron conductivity throughout the ages.

These are still the bedding materials of choice for many temperate-zone indigenous cultures around the world. Adult sleepers in traditional societies recline on skins, mats, the ground, or "just about anything except a thick, springy mattress," said a 1999 article at *Science News Online* that recommended researchers look at these societies for clues about sleeping patterns, insomnia, and nocturnal brain activity.

LIVING THINGS AS ANTENNAS

Our story brings us back to the transcendent question posed by T. H. Huxley about our relationship to Nature and the cosmos. In 1969, Matteo Tavera, a French agronomist, put forward a unique answer in the form of a series of provocative hypotheses, contained in a largely unnoticed book, in which he argued that our place on the planet was to live in accordance with "natural electricity, which governs us all." Agronomy is the application of a combination of sciences like biology, chemistry, ecology, earth science, and genetics. Tavera's commentary, drawing from all these disciplines and many years of intimately observing Nature as a farmer, concludes that humans are paying a steep price in terms of degeneration and illness as a result of their separation from Nature.

Tavera's book, published in France under the title of *La Mission Sacrée* (*The Sacred Mission*), emphasizes the unrecognized electrical relationship of all living things—including plants, animals, and humans—to the ground and sky. The Frenchman saw life on the planet as being regulated by an energizing continuum from above and below, and that our structures were designed by Nature to receive and transmit that energy. Think of our bodies and forms as antennas, he said.

Tavera lamented that the modern lifestyle included "princely like structures, all built close together . . . with isolating floors, plastic clothing, and rubber-soled shoes. The electrical contacts are slowed down or totally missing" and, as a result, an increase in chronic illness has become quite evident.

Eating more wholesome food, free of chemicals, and breathing cleaner air certainly contributes to better health. But our "sacred mission," he said, involves reconnecting with Mother Earth. Tavera warned that "man persists in going on in the direction of error," and while "Nature is forgiving, it has its limits to those who do not relate . . . and carry electricity through their bodies for the completion of the required health balance" necessary for survival.

The French naturalist said that humans should look at examples within the animal world to see why reconnection with Earth is so necessary. "Notice that a cow left in a stable with a more limited conduction of electricity due to the insulating effect of the building is usually cold and chilly," he wrote. "Put this same cow in the fields under the same weather conditions and it is quite comfortable. The cold nights are bearable. Chickens in the natural state of roaming never get sick. Chickens, isolated by their coop, need to be covered and protected . . . [and] look at the medicines that are required for the captive chicken. The quail in the wild have equal happiness in winter as in summer, without covering, without special lodging.

"The dog who is kept too long in the same habituation as his master and does not get to contact the Earth, as Nature intended, is keeping the veterinarian very busy.

"In the wild, the sanitary state of animals is excellent especially if it has not been soiled by the touch of man. Despite conditions seemingly uncomfortable to our eyes and probably because of those conditions, the wild animal knows no sickness. This privileged benefit is the result of his accomplishing his right to life by the proper exchange of the electric mediums.

"Be inspired by the wild animal [that] can survive so well on his own because of his constant contact with the Earth. Compare yourself to him a little."

Within the context of modern times, Tavera offered a variety of practical suggestions that could seemingly fit into most of our lifestyles. They included the following:

- "Walk into the wilderness and choose the grassy areas instead of the asphalt roads. Try to walk barefooted or at least with a covering that allows the electrical contact or exchange. You will notice the difference in your mood, your health. It will keep you alive with joy in your heart."

- "As often as possible expose any part of the skin of your body to the Earth or grass, or any natural water, lake, stream or ocean. In your garden . . . moist grass is a perfect conductor."

- "Use the trunk of a tree to lean on and rob it of some of its electricity for your health's benefit."

- "Bathing, especially in ocean water (because of the salts) or lake or river, is extremely good for you. If you can, walk barefoot in these waters. If you have ever done it you have already seen the benefits on your nervous system, your sleeping, your appetite, and your attitude. When you are linked to the Earth and involved in the electric exchanges, you start feeling like a human being again."

Matteo Tavera's writings are fascinating and alter the way one thinks about oneself, the environment, and our relationship with the cosmos. To read an English translation of his text on the Internet, visit the website www.earthinginstitute.net. His words offer great insight about our connectedness with Nature. What's even more fascinating is that the health implications raised by Tavera's commentary have been validated—not by a pedigreed scientist but by a non-scientist from the cable TV industry. . His personal story follows next.

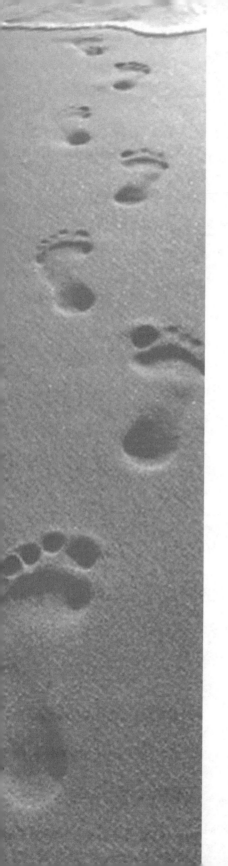

PART TWO

Personal Discoveries

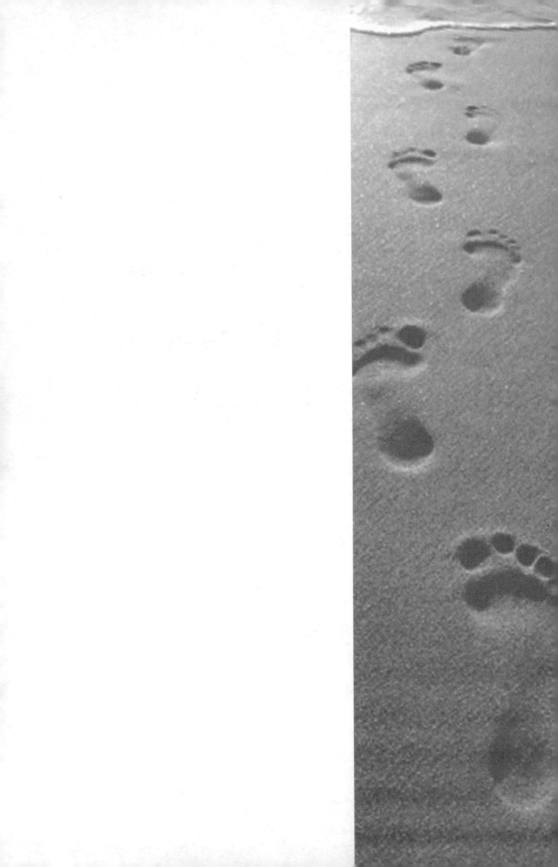

CHAPTER 3

Reconnecting: Clint Ober's Story

In 1993, I was forty-nine years old, successful, and feeling on top of the world. I had come a long way from challenging and humble beginnings as a boy who grew up on a farm, chased cows, baled hay, and spent long summer days walking barefoot up and down long rows of beets and beans pulling weeds.

When I was a teenager, my father died of leukemia, leaving my mother and six children to tend the crops and livestock. Being the eldest son, I had to drop out of school and run the family farm. This was common practice back then under those kind of circumstances.

By the early 1960s, my brothers were getting older. I felt a need to leave the land for the excitement of the "big city." I wound up in the fledgling cable television industry. In the community I lived in, we only had two TV channels—one politically right, the other politically left, so the information we got was very slanted. I quickly saw that cable was the future of television. I jumped into it enthusiastically and had a lot of success organizing marketing campaigns to bring cable to people throughout Montana. I also climbed the poles, drilled the holes, sunk the ground rods, and ran the wire to install cable systems in many homes.

After a few years of working with local cable operators, I was hired as national director of marketing for a Denver company that soon grew to become the largest cable television operator in the United States. It was eventually acquired by AT&T. In 1972, I started my own business, specializing in developing cable television systems, as well as broadcast television and microwave communication properties. The company became

27

the largest provider of cable television marketing and installation services in the country. We had a nationwide army of contract installers working for us. When a cable system was approved for some town or city, we'd send in ten to a hundred installers. They would go through the area and install everybody who wanted cable. Then they would go to the next town, and so on. Over the years we installed cable in millions of homes throughout the country.

In an age before the Internet, I helped pioneer the first-ever cable modem and distribution through personal computers of news reports from news agencies around the world. I also became intimately involved in the early development of programming and marketing for the cable and telecommunication industries. I worked with the top people who created Cable News Network (CNN), Home Box Office (HBO), and other cable networks.

I was a highly successful entrepreneur and living the good life. I had a 5,000-square-foot mountaintop home in Colorado with a 360-degree view of Denver and the Rockies. My house was full of art and anything that money could buy.

In 1993, the good life came tumbling down. I developed a serious abscess in my liver from a root canal procedure. Eighty percent of my liver was badly compromised. The infection had spread throughout my body. All my organs were malfunctioning. I didn't get much hope from the doctors. They suggested that I put my affairs in order.

However, one young surgeon told me there was a chance to survive—although a small one—involving experimental surgery to remove most of my damaged liver. He didn't give me much hope, but it was the only hope I had. So I agreed. After twenty-eight days of painful recovery in the hospital and much physical therapy, I was able to go home. I slowly began to regain my health. It took about three or four months to be able to walk a few blocks and six months to walk a mile. Amazingly, within nine months my liver grew back to its original size.

IN SEARCH OF A PURPOSE

One morning during my long mending process, I awoke and looked outside and noticed the sky was a deeper blue and the trees were a more vibrant green than I had ever seen before. At that moment, I felt alive again but very much different from before. A stark realization came over me that I didn't really own my home and the mountain of possessions I had. Rather, they owned me. My life had become all about taking care of my stuff. I'd spent my whole life accumulating, collecting, and taking care of it all, and trying to get more, perhaps to show off how big a success I was. I realized that I had become a slave to my possessions by my own making.

At that moment, I decided to set myself free and find something to fill my life with other than possessions. "I don't want anymore of this life," I said out loud to myself. "I want to do something different. Whatever time I have left I want to dedicate it to something worthwhile and with purpose."

I called my kids. They were all grown and scattered around the country. I told them to come and take whatever they wanted. "Anything you don't take, I'm going to give away," I said.

I sold the house. I sold the business to my employees. I went out and bought a recreational vehicle (RV), packed it up with a few necessities, and hit the road. I spent the next four years driving around the country, looking for myself and my mission. I spent a lot of time with my kids here and there, but a lot of time just doing nothing. I'd drive someplace and park for a while, waiting for something to show up.

One night in 1997 I was in Key Largo, Florida. I was getting antsy and impatient. Nothing was happening. Nothing was revealing itself to me. I had been in the same location now for a few months. While sitting and staring across the bay, I asked for guidance. I knew that something was waiting for me. When I returned to the RV, some words popped into my mind and I remember automatically writing them down on a piece of paper:

"Become an opposite charge."

Well, become an opposite charge to me meant to go out and poke people, and stir 'em up. Charge 'em up. I was sure getting impatient enough to do some stirring.

Then the second thing I wrote down was, "Status quo is the enemy." I didn't know what that meant except that I was getting tired of my status quo and doing nothing. That was the end of it. I wrote those thoughts down on a yellow tablet and kept it for some reason. I had no idea what those words really meant.

Upon rising the next morning, an odd notion went through my mind that the Earth itself was trying to tell me something. I didn't know what, though. But I felt there was some urgency, and I knew I had to go west somewhere for the answer. I drove to Los Angeles and felt it was too crazy. Then I drove to Tucson and Phoenix, and neither of those places felt right. So I headed north and wound up in Sedona at ten one night. I parked at a recreational vehicle resort by a creek. The next morning I looked out and was enchanted by the beauty of the land. The scenery spoke to my roots, of growing up in rural Montana, exposed to Native American culture that emphasized the connectedness to the natural world.

"I'm staying here," I told myself, "until I find what I'm looking for." So I stayed for almost two years. I made friends with many local artists and gallery owners. As a hobby, and to keep me busy, I spent a lot of my time artistically lighting up the town's many art galleries.

My "lightbulb" went off one day in 1998. I was sitting on a park bench and watching the passing parade of tourists from all over the world. At some point, and I don't know why, my awareness zeroed in on what all these different people were wearing on their feet. I saw a lot of those running shoes with thick rubber or plastic soles. I was wearing them as well. It occurred to me rather innocently that all these people—me included—were insulated from the ground, the electrical surface charge of the Earth beneath our feet. I started to think about static electricity and wondered if being insulated like that could have some effect on health. I didn't know the answer, one way or another. The notion just popped into my mind.

I thought back to my years in television and cable. Before there was cable, you commonly had lots of flecks ("noise," we call it) in the TV picture. Or you had "snow" or lines and all kinds of electromagnetic interference. If you aren't old enough to remember that, you are likely familiar with the radio interference when you're driving near or under a power line and you hear all that crackle and pop.

In the cable industry, you have to ground and shield the entire cable system in every home to prevent extraneous electromagnetic signals and fields from interfering with the transmission carried through the cable.

That's how you provide the viewer with a perfect signal and a crisp picture, as well as preventing signals on the cable system from leaking out into the environment and possibly disturbing police radio or TV station transmissions. The cable consists of an inner copper conductor, an insulating layer, and an outer shield. The shield is electrically connected to the Earth. It is grounded, so that the Earth can either deliver or absorb electrons and prevent damage from electrical charges. All of the cable system must be grounded and held at the same electrical potential as the Earth's surface.

What Is Electrostatic Discharge?

Static electricity is nothing more than the spark or minor shock we all experience, for instance, when we touch a metal doorknob after walking across a carpeted room (see figure below) or slide across a car seat. No big deal.

But in some industries, it is a very big deal. Centuries ago, armed forces had to use static control measures to prevent ignition of gunpowder stores. Today, such measures are required in the petroleum industry, where a random spark can also cause an explosion. In today's electronic industry, electrostatic discharge (ESD) causes billions of dollars in damage annually by destroying highly sensitive electronic parts and microchips. ESD affects production yields, manufacturing costs, product quality, product reliability, and profitability.

A whole static control industry has emerged with products such as wristbands, shoes, and conductive flooring that are widely used by electronics makers. These measures are designed to discharge potentially destructive charges.

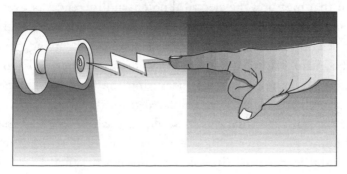

Finger to the doorknob, showing electrostatic discharge.

THE BEGINNING OF AN ADVENTURE

Little did I know at the time, but my life was about to take a new and totally unexpected direction that would consume practically all my waking hours. It still continues to do so, a dozen years later.

It all started innocently with that one simple question: Could wearing rubber- or plastic-soled shoes, as we all do, and insulating ourselves from the ground, affect health? At the time I had a particular interest in health because earlier back surgeries had left me with constant back pain. I never slept well. I'd take Advil to go to bed, and in the morning I'd take Advil to get up and get through the day. I also took other pain medication, depending on how bad the pain was.

I knew that the body was conductive, that is, it conducts electricity. You don't have to know anything about electricity to understand that simple fact of life. Just go touch a doorknob on a very dry day and you can see or feel a spark every time. There's always a static charge on the body that builds up when you sit on fabric-covered furniture or walk on carpets.

An Amazing Experiment

Sitting there watching the foot traffic I realized that most people, certainly in the industrialized world, had little or no connection to the ground. In other parts of the world, like in the tropics and in Asia, Africa, and South America, rural people walk barefoot and often sleep on the ground. They are grounded.

I decided to try to answer the question I had asked myself. I went back to the apartment I was renting and picked up my voltmeter. (A voltmeter is an instrument that measures the electrical potential differences between the Earth and any electrical object, or any two points in an electrical circuit.) I connected a 50-foot wire to it and ran the wire out the living room door and attached it to a simple ground rod I stuck in the Earth. Then I started walking around the house and measuring the electrical charges being created on my body from being insulated from the ground. It was easy to measure the static electricity, as it would vary with every step that I took. What I found most interesting was the amount of electromagnetic field (EMF) induced potential (in volts) on my body. When I walked toward a lamp, the voltage would go up. When I stepped back, the voltage went down. I tested this with all the electrical appliances in the living room and kitchen. The only appliances that did not create EMF voltage on my body were the refrigerator and my computer tower. They were grounded. From my background in the communications industry, this immediately made sense to me as we had to ground all of our electronic equipment to prevent electrical interference from EMFs.

Next I went to the bedroom, lay down on my bed, and registered the highest level of EMF voltage on my body. The bedroom was the most "electrically active" area of the apartment. The bed was up against a wall full of hidden electrical wires. I wondered if these electric fields could be affecting my ability to fall asleep because sleep was always a big problem.

Now my curiosity was really stirred up. The next day I went to the hardware store and bought some metallized duct tape that is used for furnace ducting. I laid some of that tape out on the bed to form a crude kind of grid. I took an alligator clip and attached it to one end of the duct tape grid. I connected a wire to it, ran the wire out the window, and fastened it to another ground rod similar to the one that the voltmeter was connected to. I then lay down on the duct tape grid and noticed that the meter was now showing nearly zero, meaning that I was in sync, that is electrically equivalent, to lying directly on the ground outside. Like all the cable systems I had installed, I was physically grounded. I was lying there fooling around with the voltmeter and the next thing I knew it was morning. I had fallen asleep with the voltmeter on my chest. I hadn't needed a pill to fall asleep. I had slept soundly for the first time in years, and I had hardly moved at all during the night.

"Wow, this is fascinating," I said to myself. Something interesting had happened, but I didn't really understand the meaning of it. So I repeated this experiment on myself the next night. I fell asleep without a pill. The same thing happened the next night and the next and the next.

Getting High Off the Ground

After a few more days like this, I told a couple of friends about it and asked them if I could set up a similar kind of makeshift grid with metallic duct tape in their beds. That's how I started "grounding" people. It was very innocent. One of the guys I grounded said to me, "You know, something is going on here. My arthritis pain is way down."

I didn't think too much about what he said, but a couple of days later I noticed that my own severe chronic pain had improved. I didn't need the pain pills anymore. I was also feeling much better overall.

I didn't understand anything about biology. I didn't understand how the nerves or muscles worked, but a concept was dawning. It occurred to me that there might be an analogy between the human body and cable TV. Cable has hundreds of channels of information flowing through it. Similarly, the body has countless nerves, blood vessels, and other channels that conduct electrical signals. Maybe, I thought, when the body is grounded, it prevents the entry of "noise"—environmental electrical interference—that could disturb the internal circuitry. I started to understand in a simple way that without Earth contact the body was always being charged by the electromagnetic fields and static electricity in the bedroom or office or wherever. When you're grounded, you don't have a charge. When I grounded myself and my friends, the charges were removed, and we all started sleeping better and feeling better.

After I grounded a half dozen or so people, consistently improving their sleep and reducing their pain, I started to get a real high. I became more and more excited. I came to the conclusion that I may have made a great discovery. I said to myself there's something very, very real here that needs to be further investigated.

I looked far and wide but didn't find much information on grounding and health. In 1999, the Internet wasn't nearly the information universe it is today. It was still fairly new and I didn't find anything there.

I checked out the excellent university medical libraries in Arizona but didn't come up with anything. There were a few anecdotal stories about Native Americans that were folklorish in nature. I was reminded of my younger days in Montana where many of my childhood friends were kids from the Indian reservation. I vividly remembered the time when the sister of one of my friends developed a bad case of scarlet fever. She was very sick. Their grandfather dug a pit in the ground and placed the girl in the pit. He built a fire, for warmth, near the pit, and sat next to it for a few days while the girl mostly slept. At the end of that time she was much better. I also remembered going to the home of one of my friends after school and hearing his mother tell him to remove his shoes. "They will make you sick," she said. This all seemed very odd to me at the time, but I remembered that most things the Native Americans did were different from what I was taught to be normal. I later realized that there was always a reason based on much greater knowledge of Nature than I was ever taught.

I found information about barefoot enthusiasts who have long championed the idea of going unshod because they feel better. Some enthusiasts have formed organizations, such as the worldwide Society for Barefoot Living that promotes the benefits of taking shoes and socks off and walking naturally on the Earth. Their experience, along with medical research in the field of biomechanics, strongly suggests that many foot and back problems are partly caused by stresses and strains created by wearing shoes that force us to stand and move in ways the human body was not designed for. One dramatic example of this appears to be the success of barefoot runners. The shod foot may explain the high injury frequency in North American runners, in contrast to the extremely low running-related injury frequency in barefoot populations. Researchers have found, for instance, less force on the joints, and less plantar fasciitis and shin splints. This, however, wasn't really the information I was looking for.

I did find considerable information about electrostatic discharge and how people working on computer components and electronic chips had to be grounded in order not to damage any of the components electrically. But that wasn't it either. I had to keep looking.

I also wanted to know whether there was any possibility that sleeping "Earthed," as I started to call grounding, could be harmful. Electronics experts reassured me that the concept was perfectly safe. If you think about it, being Earthed is the natural state of living systems throughout history. It is the separation from Earth that is unnatural.

Beyond these few things, however, I couldn't uncover any concrete information anywhere relating to the possible health effects due to loss of natural grounding.

CHAPTER 4

Challenges of an Amateur Scientist

Emotionally, I was on a roller coaster. I came to the conclusion that nobody—past or present—had researched the grounding/health connection. I couldn't find any relevant information. When I realized that nobody else knew about it, I felt it was like the best day in my life and that I had discovered something important with which to help society in a big way. I had found my mission. And I was the only one who knew anything about it.

The euphoria didn't last long. Maybe that's the way it is with discoveries. The self-doubt starts to creep in that comes from being alone with some important understanding or breakthrough before anybody accepts your idea.

In my case, anybody who I talked to thought I was nuts. Nobody took me seriously. Nobody knew anything. My enthusiasm would always be returned by blank stares of indifference or negative responses. Who said this was so? People wanted hard facts. They wanted science. I was just an ex-cable guy talking about how the ground could reduce your pain and let you sleep better. What did I know? What credentials did I have?

So I went quickly from the best day in my life to the worst day. I was feeling down in the dumps one day in 1999 as I was sitting and talking with one of the guys in Sedona whom I'd grounded. He was telling me how good he felt and how big the change was in his life. Hearing him say those words reignited a spark and lifted my spirits.

I said to him, "I'm feeling good from this, too. Other people are telling me the same thing. This is real. I'm not making anything up. There's no ifs, ands, or buts about it. I've just got to find the answers."

With new resolve, I packed up and drove to California in my RV, an amateur detective trying to solve a mystery. I figured I'd spend a few months out there and hopefully turn up some real expertise that I could tap into, some people to teach me more, or to figure out how to quantify what all this was about.

"STRANGER IN A STRANGE LAND"

The first thing I did was try to interest sleep researchers in Southern California. I made phone calls. I knocked on doors. I introduced myself as a guy with an electrical background who has made some interesting observations about sleep and pain. I had seen dramatic results. I said I wanted to get some experts to validate my observations.

In pursuit of expertise, I felt like the hero of Robert Heinlein's old science fiction classic, *Stranger in a Strange Land*. I felt I was on another planet. I didn't speak the language. They didn't speak mine.

Imagine how I felt walking into the office of a scientist or doctor, if I got that far. The office walls were full of awards and diplomas. These were individuals who had spent years becoming experts in their field. And here I was, with absolutely no formal training in the field. The experts used biological terms I never heard of. When I would turn the conversation to electrical concepts that I understood, like voltages, electric fields, grounding, and positive and negative charges in the body, they were about as clueless as I was hearing them talk about what they knew.

Communication was just one problem. Another was that most scientists or doctors had no desire to get involved or lend their name to anything out of left field like this, something with no scientific history or legitimacy.

One scientist sat back and laughed in my face. He asked if I expected him "to believe that sticking a nail in the ground and connecting it to an iron bed pad and getting people to sleep on it will reduce pain." He said he wouldn't believe it even if it were published in the *New England Journal of Medicine*.

One doctor told me that even if what I was saying were true, why should he tell patients to take off their shoes and get well for free?

Another stated that I needed to provide him with all the published research related to grounding the body and he would then take a look at it. When I told him there was no research and that is why I was approaching him, he said to come back after someone substantiates the validity of grounding.

One amused researcher asked if I had any idea about what it takes to do research. He told me it would take five years and $5 million to put together a real scientific study and get it published, if it even got that far.

Most of the experts I spoke to were polite, but nobody took any interest. They sent me on my way and wished me good luck. That's when I decided to do the first study myself.

GETTING THE SCIENCE BALL ROLLING

All wasn't lost though. At one university sleep clinic, I managed to talk to some friendly students. They said they would be willing to counsel me how to do a study. I didn't have a clue. One thing I had to figure out was how I could ground people for any length of time, long enough so that I could identify a measurable result. People are always moving around. They are busy.

So I went back to my own experience. The only way to do this, I realized, was when somebody was in bed, at night, when sleeping. That's the only time people are still. That seemed to be the most practical way to produce a measurement. So a bed pad of some sort seemed the best way to go. But I had to design something more substantial than the crude metallic duct tape grid I was using for myself and friends.

I contacted a company that makes protective equipment for the electronics industry. I had some special conductive fiber materials manufactured that I then bonded to 1-by-2-foot wool felt pads. The test subjects were to sleep directly on the pad placed on their bed. I fixed a metallic snap on each pad so I could connect it to a wire running to a ground rod stuck in the Earth outside the bedroom window. Now that I had a pad, I needed people for the experiment.

As you can imagine, no doctors would lend me patients for my little study. I was on my own. I got the inspiration for volunteers one day while getting my hair cut. I heard people in the salon talking about their health issues. I figured that a beauty salon could be a good source of volunteers. I convinced the woman who operated the salon to try grounding first. I set her up with a grounded bed pad. Her feedback was positive. She was sleeping better. She enthusiastically approached some of her clients to participate in the study. I found others by leaving fliers in ten beauty shops in Ventura, California, where I was living at the time.

One of the people who stepped forward was a nurse. She was a great help, smoothing the way so I could enter the homes of strangers, explain the bed pads, actually place them in people's beds, and connect them to simple ground rods I stuck in the Earth outside their bedroom windows. What I was doing was not exactly your ordinary house call. In the end, I was able to enroll sixty people—thirty-eight women and twenty-two men—with sleep problems and a variety of joint and muscle pain.

Based on the advice I had received from the sleep clinic students, I divided the volunteers into two groups. Half slept on pads that were actually grounded. For comparison, the other half slept on bed pads that looked like they were connected to the ground rods, but I inserted a spacer on the wire to block conduction. The volunteers did not know if they were actually connected or not. I was the only one who knew.

The nurse interacted with the people during the thirty days' experiment. Then she collected the data. We then wrote up the experiment as an anecdotal study and published it in 2000 on *ESD,* an online journal that provides articles, technical papers, news items, and book reviews on the subject of electrostatics.

The results were extraordinary. Here is what we found afterward when we compared the grounded group with the ungrounded one:

- 85 percent went to sleep more quickly.

- 93 percent reported sleeping better throughout the night.

- 82 percent experienced a significant reduction in muscle stiffness.

- 74 percent experienced elimination or reduction of chronic back and joint pain.

- 100 percent reported feeling more rested when they woke up.

- 78 percent reported improved general health.

Several participants reported unexpected but significant relief from asthmatic and respiratory conditions, rheumatoid arthritis, hypertension (high blood pressure), sleep apnea, and premenstrual syndrome (PMS). There were also reports of fewer hot flashes.

Discovery of the "Magic Pain Patch"

One woman who participated in the study had crippling rheumatoid arthritis in the joints of her hands and arms, and she had difficulty walking. I wanted to measure how much electrical charge she had on her body in her bedroom and asked her to hold a small, handheld tester for me. She couldn't. Her arthritis was too severe and too painful. So in order to get a reading I adhered an electrode patch—the same kind used by doctors when they do EKG (electrocardiogram) tests—on her forearm and connected it with an alligator clip to the ground wire coming into her bedroom. I then connected and disconnected the clip in order to read the change in the body charge between being grounded and ungrounded. After chatting for five or ten minutes while I was setting up the bed-pad system, the woman said the pain in her arm improved considerably. She then asked me to move the patch to her other arm. I did not believe what she was saying, but I did what she asked and moved the patch to the other arm. Minutes later, she said the pain in that arm had gone down a good deal as well.

After leaving her home, I immediately called several acquaintances I knew who had arthritis and other painful conditions, and gave them each setups with electrode patches, Earthing wires, and ground rods. I wanted to see if I could repeat this dramatic reduction of localized pain. Remarkably, each and every one of them reported a rapid reduction in pain. A couple of them referred to it as the "magic pain patch." This is when I first discovered that localized Earthing of the body in this manner produced fast and dramatic reduction of local pain. It was kind of like pouring water on a fire.

Now I was really excited. I felt encouraged. But still no scientists would talk to me seriously about it. My student buddies told me that I needed to produce much more solid information to support my idea. Anecdotal studies wouldn't be enough, they said, and wouldn't stand up to scientific scrutiny.

Refining the Discovery

Initially I regarded the positive results I was witnessing as a consequence of eliminating static electricity and/or the shielding of the body from environmental electric fields. This assumption turned out to be absolutely true, but accounted only in part for all the good results.

When I installed the Earthing system in people's homes for the first study, I always measured their body voltages while they were lying in bed—both before and after placing the grounding pad on the bed. When I measured people with extremely high body voltage, I would think to myself that I should get some really good results from this person.

One day I set up a volunteer, a sixty-five-year-old man, who complained of chronic pain and problems with sleeping. He had no electrical devices near the bed. His floor was bare concrete. When I measured his body voltage, it registered near zero. With very little body voltage, I thought we wouldn't get any results from him. However, his feedback in the end was as good as others with high body voltages.

His case was the first indication I had that Earthing alone produced the results that I myself had experienced and observed in others. This realization stopped me in my tracks. I then had to learn everything I could about the Earth's electrical properties.

I learned, for instance, that the Earth's electrical surface charge is always negative, meaning that the surface is filled with free electrons. They are able to move and reduce a positive charge. In Nature, lightning is the best example of a negative charge reducing a positive charge.

If Earthing people reduces their chronic pain, that suggested to me that pain is related to positive charge. I then began to ground people in low- or no-electric field environments to replicate this observation and confirm that it was the grounding alone that reduced pain. The results were consistent. Earthing reduced pain no matter what the electrical environment. It wasn't until later that I learned the connection between chronic pain and inflammation, and the role of electrons.

NORMALIZING THE HORMONE OF STRESS

When the first study was published, it created a big stir among researchers and health practitioners concerned about the health risks from exposure to environmental electric fields. One such person I met at this time was Maurice Ghaly, a retired anesthesiologist in Southern California who was interested in electric field research. I told him what I had learned. He pretty much dismissed my theory. But he said he would like to prove me wrong. It didn't make sense to him that grounding could do what I said it did.

Dr. Ghaly decided on a pilot study. He would measure the circadian secretion of cortisol on people before and after they slept grounded, over a period of a few weeks. Cortisol is known as the "stress hormone." When you become worried, fearful, and anxious, your cortisol level rises. The rise stimulates a branch of the autonomic nervous system known as the sympathetic system. Your body shifts into a vigilant mode, ready, if needed, to fight or run, the so-called fight-or-flight mode. The hormone level comes back down after the vigilance and tension ease. A life of constant stress—from common things like money, work, or relationship problems—also causes your cortisol level to rise and remain high, creating a kind of sympathetic overdrive in the body. In our day and age, a consistently high level is a classic indicator of stress and is known to contribute to many health problems, like sleep disorders, hypertension, cardiovascular disease, reduced immune response, autoimmune disease, mood disturbances, and blood sugar irregularity. Stress of this kind also promotes inflammation in the body.

My first study was subjective, based on the feedback of people I grounded. This time we would measure a substance produced in the body, thus providing an objective measurement for the effect of Earthing on the physiology. It was a big step forward scientifically.

For the study, I needed something that would hold up even better than the previous bed pad. So I designed a sturdier bed pad that would fit over the whole mattress.

We enrolled twelve subjects who complained of sleep problems, pain, and stress. They slept on the Earthing pads I made up for eight weeks. Their individual daily cortisol levels were determined at four-hour intervals over a twenty-four hour period just before the start of the study and then once again at the three-quarter mark via a standard saliva test. The participants also reported daily how they were feeling throughout the entire experiment.

The study was published in a 2004 issue of the *Journal of Alternative and Complementary Medicine*. The conclusion was significant: Earthing during sleep resynchronizes cortisol secretion more in alignment with its natural, normal rhythm—highest at 8:00 a.m. and lowest at midnight. Figure 4-1 provides a visual representation of the dramatically improved cortisol group profile.

Cortisol levels before and after grounding

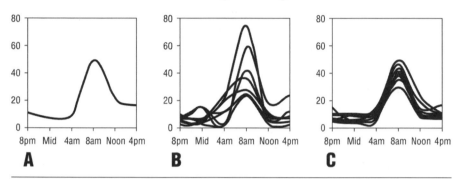

Figure 4-1. Realignment of natural cortisol rhythms.

In unstressed individuals, the normal twenty-four-hour cortisol secretion profile follows a predictable pattern—lowest around 12:00 midnight and highest at 8:00 a.m. (Graph A). The pre-grounding chart (Graph B) shows the wide variation of patterns among the study participants. Graph C represents the altered pattern of the participants after Earthing, showing a significant stabilization of cortisol levels. Seven participants registered a reduction in high- to out-of-range nighttime cortisol secretion, a 53.7 percent average drop; six had an average rise towards normal of 34.3 percent in 8:00 a.m. levels; and two with abnormally high 8:00 a.m. levels had an average drop of 38 percent. (Data adapted from *The Journal of Alternative and Complementary Medicine, 2004.*)

Subjectively, the participants reported improved sleep along with reduced pain and stress. Even more impressive was the fact that the improvements often occurred within the very first days of sleeping grounded.

Following is a summary of the findings:

• All but two subjects developed more natural cortisol rhythm, and one of the exceptions was someone already in a normal pattern.

• Eleven of twelve participants said they fell asleep faster.

- All twelve reported waking fewer times during the night (from an average of 2.5 times to 1.4 times, a 44 percent reduction).

- Nine out of twelve said they felt more refreshed and less fatigued, with more daytime energy, while three reported no change.

- Of the eleven subjects who said before grounding that their pain interfered with general activities, seven now reported improvement and only four said there was no change.

- Nine out of twelve described reductions in their emotional stress and were less bothered by problems such as anxiety, depression, and irritability; two said there was no change; one said the stress was worse.

- Six out of seven participants reported improvements of gastrointestinal symptoms.

- Five out of six women with either PMS and/or hot flashes said their symptoms were better,

- All three individuals with TMJ (temporomandibular joint) pain said their discomfort was less.

The Sleep Connection

The study produced another quite interesting finding that was not published but provided more evidence about the multiple benefits of Earthing. Eight of our participants had an increase in melatonin ranging from 2 to 16 percent. Three subjects had no change in their melatonin level, and one experienced a decrease of 6 percent. The finding was exciting because melatonin is an important hormone that helps regulate sleep and other biological rhythms and is also a powerful antioxidant agent with anti-cancer properties.

Right from the start of my experimenting with Earthing—and by right from the start I mean my own initial experience—the positive impact on sleep has been very noticeable. This is a big deal. We all need good rest to allow our bodies to repair and recover from each day's activities. That's the way Nature set things up: cycles of rest and activity.

After I saw how grounding was helping people sleep, I started to research the sleep problem. I found a 2002 *Newsweek* article entitled "In Search of Sleep" that said there were an estimated 70 million problem sleepers in the United States alone. "I Can't Sleep" was the title of a *BusinessWeek* cover story in 2004. From those, and many other sleep-related articles from all over the world, it became quite clear to me that quality sleep improves overall health and that poor sleep does just the opposite.

I also learned that back in the early 1970s researchers identified several behaviors that were positively linked to length of life. Sleep headed the list, followed by exercise, eating breakfast, and avoiding snacks. Weight, smoking, and moderating alcohol intake also made the list. Later on, researchers found that sleep deprivation may enable bacterial growth and that sufficient sleep may slow down bacterial growth. More recently, sleep deprivation—even a modest reduction—was found to promote inflammation in the body. Loss of sleep, even for a few short hours during the night, apparently prompts the immune system to turn against healthy tissue and organs. Other new studies suggest that sleep loss may also contribute to recurrent depression.

In my ongoing sleuthing, I learned that since the pioneering research in the 1950s of Hans Selye, the father of stress medicine, medical researchers believe there is a relationship between imbalances in cortisol and inflammatory pain.

It was becoming clearer and clearer to me that Earthing was something very special that could make people's lives better in a multitude of ways. It was this vision that kept me going, because there were many times when I frankly felt overwhelmed by the challenge of me—an unknown quantity with no degree by my name, or even a high school education—proving a totally foreign concept to the scientific community.

MORE CHALLENGES: BEDS, SPOUSES, AND FASHION

My first sleep study created a buzz when it was published in 2000. I was hounded by people wanting bed pads. All of a sudden, there was a demand for this "quasi product." I didn't realize it at the time, but I was becoming somewhat of a designer of Earthing pads. Later, when I got involved in Earthing people in the world of sports, athletes didn't want a whole bed pad. It was too much to carry around. They wanted something they could roll up and put in a small bag and take with them when they traveled. Thus, the recovery bag was born: conductive silver strands woven into cotton sheets fitted together like a sleeping bag.

The products developed both out of a demand by people who heard about Earthing as well as a desire on my part to promote scientific research. It all started on an ad-lib basis with conductive duct tape and a wire connection to a ground rod. That's what I used in Arizona on myself, friends, and other interested people. It was all makeshift. Nothing sophisticated.

As this evolved, people simply wanted something more refined. Some people wanted sheets, so I started consulting with experts in the fabric industry. I first dabbled in polyester with carbon threads. But nobody wanted polyester, so I switched to cotton with conductive silver strands. That development cost more than $1 million and took three to four years. I first had to find manufacturers to deal with what for them was a nuisance factor, and then test and retest. These were all prototype products that cost a lot of money to make, and for the most part, I was giving them away to athletes, doctors, and people in the studies and their relatives. It all mushroomed. I would get rid of one model, then order more, then get another batch of new material, and then another flurry of orders and requests. I never for a moment thought I would be in the sleeping or bedding industry.

In the early days, a lot of doctors started getting products for their patients. One of them called and asked if I had some kind of a "half pad," a sheet that didn't cover the whole bed. I asked why he wanted it. He referred to the spouse problem.

Spouse problem?

Here is what was going on: If a woman got a bed pad, the husband would get upset and say he didn't want anything to do with this, that it was just a waste of money. If the husband brought it home, the woman would say this is crazy and get it off her side of the bed.

Throughout this time, the mode of the day was to put sheets on your bed with the highest possible thread count. The buzz was 300-, 600-, 1,200-, and then 2,400-count sheets. The higher the count, the more luxurious, softer, and finer the fabric is supposed to be. This concept became very popular, but some experts think that higher thread counts simply mean a higher price tag.

Anyway, I got caught up in this. If you had anything else but high thread count on your bed, you were not in fashion. Then there was the issue of designer colors to match décor and color tastes. In a typical marriage, nothing goes on a bed without a woman's permission. So you couldn't put just anything on a bed—no matter what the health benefits.

I didn't need these kinds of extraneous issues. One day I decided to just make a half sheet that could be placed across the width of the bottom of the bed. You make contact with it with your feet, like putting your feet on the Earth, and this is your barefoot connection. The half sheet could also be used lengthwise on one side if a spouse didn't want to have anything to do with it.

The half sheet solved a lot of my headaches, as well as reducing the pain level for many people who slept on them.

CHAPTER 5

A Cardiologist's Discovery: Steve Sinatra's Story

As an integrative cardiologist, I use both conventional and alternative medicine to help my cardiac patients. This approach has always worked superbly for me as a doctor and, above all, for my patients, because it focuses on the metabolic operation of cells and particularly the cells in the heart muscle that pump blood throughout the sixty thousand miles of blood vessels in the body. As such, I have used many excellent nutritional supplements, like coenzyme Q10 (CoQ10), carnitine, and magnesium, to boost the metabolic processes in the cells where energy production takes place.

Years ago, after a decade or so in practice, I slowly became aware of a curious pattern: increased patient complaints—notably arrhythmias and chest pain (angina)—around the time of a full moon or intensified solar flare activity. I don't remember how I actually connected the symptoms with celestial events—it may have been a patient who said something. I certainly had no real clue how to explain it. In any case, my curiosity was tweaked and I began looking for information, which led me into the amazing world of electromedicine.

The term may sound way out in left field and conjure images of Dr. Frankenstein, Dr. Sivana, Goldfinger, and otherworldly contraptions that snap, crackle, and pop. However, electromedicine is quite an accepted concept, most obviously for diagnostics that includes everyday medical tools such as EKGs and MRIs (magnetic resonance images). Less accepted, but gaining increased medical attention and respect, are electromagnetic treatment devices such as pulsed electromagnetic field units to address pain and musculoskeletal disorder. Pain-reducing TENS (transcutaneous electrical nerve stimulation) machines, utilizing low electrical voltage, have been around for many years.

My research and conversations with experts has given me a growing understanding as to how electromagnetic events going on in the heavens or right here on the planet can have a response—positive or negative—on the heart, the brain, and the rest of the body. For sure, we terrestrials are not isolated from the rest of the universe and are subject to influences ranging from galactic and solar forces down to local, man-made electricity and electronics.

All beings are conglomerations of bioelectrical energy. In essence, our bodies function—for better or for worse—as a collection of dynamic electrical circuits.

One of the primary electrical entities in the body is the heart. Each beat is triggered by an electrical signal from within the heart muscle, activity that is recorded when you undergo an EKG in your doctor's office. Each signal, repeated nonstop during a lifetime, passes through cardiac circuitry, causing the heart to contract and push blood through the chambers and then out into your body.

Heart disease can disrupt this normal electrical and pumping operation. For instance, problems with the electrical system—known as arrhythmias—can make it difficult for the heart to pump blood efficiently. Because of the electrical nature of the heart, it was natural for a curious cardiologist like me to be attracted to energy and electrical concepts that might affect the cardiovascular system in some beneficial way.

In 2001, I was invited to speak at an electromedicine conference in San Diego. That's where I met Clint Ober. He had just completed his second study—how grounding affected cortisol and stress—and he was interested in discussing his research with a cardiologist who had an interest in electromedicine. He looked me up at the conference. We talked awhile, and I was immediately intrigued by his concept. Afterward, we met in his RV and talked in more detail. There was another medical doctor present, as well as a researcher who had developed a cuff to measure blood vessel elasticity. The researcher had his device with him and he used it to test our individual elasticity. You want your arteries to be good and elastic. Rigid, constricted blood vessels are symptomatic of high blood pressure and arterial disease. My reading was good, but Clint's was enviously better. He was about two years older than me, so I was very impressed. I remember thinking how could this guy have a better result than me? Here I was, the big prevention doctor who wrote books and newsletters about healthy lifestyle!

Clint said in his usual soft-spoken voice that he believed the results had to do with the fact that he grounded himself all the time. He slept grounded, and he walked barefoot whenever possible.

Clint also shared with me his frustration with the medical and scientific community that had shown little or no interest in grounding. He was having a hard time getting a foot inside the door of science.

A NEW HEALING FRONTIER

If anything, I felt like a door to a new healing frontier had been pulled open by the most unlikely of individuals. Over my decades of practicing medicine, I had heard countless inspiring talks from the greatest and most honored medical experts. Doctors. Scientists. Professors. Nobel Prize winners. Clint Ober was none of those. He said he was "just" a cable TV guy who had made a discovery he felt could help alleviate suffering. I was impressed by his integrity and intentions. He was somebody with a mission. I felt he was on to something very important and fundamental, with great potential not just for cardiology, but also for the healing community at large. He had just a bare beginning of scientific evidence to back up his observations. Nevertheless, as a cardiologist, it made a lot of sense to me. In addition, my intuition was telling me this was big and exciting and on the mark.

For years, I had been doing a lot of research and writing about antioxidants. In my cardiac practice, I had found that antioxidant nutritional supplements, such as CoQ10, gave a clinically significant healing boost to my patients. I was curious as to whether there was an antioxidant and inflammation connection to Clint's discovery.

Just a year or so before, Harvard researchers had published strong evidence to show that chronic inflammation was a leading cause of arterial disease that chokes off blood, nutrients, and oxygen to the heart and brain, resulting in heart attacks and stroke.

So inflammation and antioxidants were on my mind when I met Clint. I asked him about inflammation. Could grounding reduce inflammation? If it did, grounding might represent a new weapon against heart disease, the No. 1 disease killer in America, and many other common conditions linked to inflammation.

I didn't know the answer. Clint didn't know.

I asked if he could find out.

He said he would. And he did, pretty much on his own at first, and later with the help of a terrific biophysicist, James Oschman.

EARTH/BODY MEDICINE

Clint, with his knowledge of electricity and grounding cable TV systems, now began to exhaustively study physiology and the immune system. He quickly began putting two and two together. Electrical engineers knew that the surface of the Earth is pulsating with negative-charged free electrons. Medical scientists didn't know that, but they did know that the body is electrical in nature, and that free radicals are positive-charged molecules at the core of inflammation, tissue destruction, and disease. Clint theorized that if Earthing reduces pain, it must come from reducing or neutralizing the positive-charged free radicals causing the pain during the inflammatory process. The free electrons must be putting out the fire.

Clint called me one day, excited about having found another important explanation for how grounding was working in the body. It didn't "just" normalize cortisol, improve sleep, and reduce stress, as if those weren't enough. If somebody is in direct contact with the Earth—barefoot or through one of his grounded pads—the free electrons flow into the conductive circuitry of the body and snuff out inflammation. Inflammation causes pain. People with pain who are grounded experience less pain.

For him, the connection was simple.

Get grounded.

Get well.

Get pain relief.

Heal.

People talk about mind/body medicine. I've been practicing that for years. I never heard anybody talk about earth/body medicine before Clint.

To me, this was another landmark finding, a major breakthrough. This was literally electromedicine from the ground up. A secret of the ages right under my feet. For me, the original anti-inflammatory and the ultimate antioxidant had been found.

SLEEPING AND FISHING GROUNDED

After meeting Clint, I had obtained one of his prototype mattress pads and started sleeping grounded. The difference was profound. My wife and I were both able to fall asleep faster. I still use that same pad to this day. I wrote about sleeping grounded in my health newsletter in 2002, and a number of my subscribers obtained a bed pad for themselves. Some took the time to give me feedback afterward and said it had made a difference in their lives.

In time, as I became involved in some of Clint's research projects and heard the feedback from people whose heart functions had improved, the exciting potential of Earthing as a tool against heart disease started to crystallize.

I travel a good deal, giving lectures and attending medical conferences, and sleeping in hotels has always been problematic. Later on, when Clint designed some portable models, we were able to sleep grounded on the road just as we did at home. Now I never leave home without my pad, and I'm always looking for opportunities to walk barefoot.

For years, I used to suffer with flare-ups of psoriasis, a common inflammatory condition of the skin. It would appear on my lower legs and elbows. I had always noticed that whenever I would go bonefishing off the Florida coast—a favorite recreational pursuit of mine—the psoriasis would virtually disappear for weeks afterward. I attributed that to the healing influence of being out in the sun, the vitamin D, the minerals in the salt water, and time off from the daily stresses of a busy cardiology practice. In bonefishing, you spend hours casting for fish with a fly rod while walking on white sand flats knee-deep in crystal clear water. After meeting Clint, I realized that there was another reason for the improvement of the psoriasis. I was grounded, barefoot in salt water that is highly conductive. As I was fishing, I was simultaneously giving myself a treatment. Now that I ground myself at night, the psoriasis is virtually gone.

Bob Tolve, an old fishing buddy of mine from Scarsdale, New York, shared an interesting story with me after I told him about Earthing. Bob is sixty-three, my age, and has been in the construction business for many years. When he started out as a young man, he worked for a while with a crew of older carpenters from Norway. He recalled them telling him that if he wanted to last in the business he should do as they do: first thing in the morning go out and walk barefoot on the wet Earth. That would take away the aches and pains of the profession, they said. Bob never forgot the story.

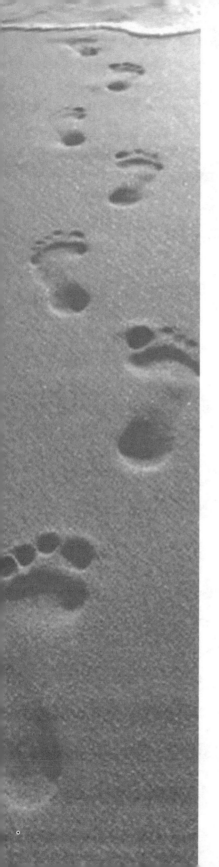

PART THREE

Connecting
with Science

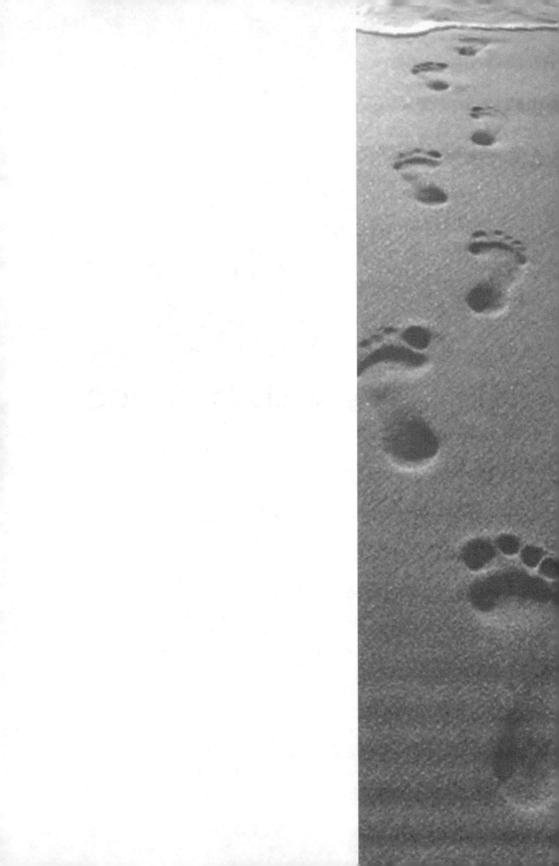

CHAPTER 6

The Original Anti-Inflammatory

The Earth itself is the original anti-inflammatory. And the planet itself is the biggest electron donor on the planet.

What does this mean to you?

Just imagine negative-charged electrons, like a mighty unseen cavalry, galloping up through your body from the Earth and mopping up an outnumbered force of positive-charged inflammatory free radicals. Electron deficiency, created by a lack of grounding, is eliminated and a healing process unfolds.

The inflammation, sickness, and pain in your body are but a manifestation—in large part or small—of an electron deficiency. The remedy is as close as the Earth you live on.

In 2000, Clint Ober was asked by a friend if he would ground an elderly gentleman who was bedridden with advanced rheumatoid arthritis. The man's hands, elbows, and feet were grotesquely misshapen and inflamed. He was racked with pain and could hardly move and then only very slowly. He was receiving comfort and at-home support from hospice, the national organization that offers services to patients whose life expectancy is six months or less.

Ober said he would come and see what could be done. It took three people to lift the man out of the bed in order to allow a conductive bed pad to be placed on it. The pad was then connected to a ground rod outside.

About ten days later, Ober received a phone call from the man, asking if he could come over again. He said that a squirrel had eaten through the ground wire.

"How do you know that?" Ober wanted to know.

"I went out and saw it had been chewed through," the man said.

Ober was puzzled. How could a bedridden patient be up and about in his yard in a matter of a few days?

"That's what I did," he said. "I went out and saw it."

Astonished, Ober drove up again. He found the man waiting for him, leaning against the front door. He said he was feeling better. And he was right about the wire. It had indeed been chewed up by an animal. Ober replaced it.

After the elderly patient had used the bed pad for a year, Ober learned from his friend that the man was much improved. He was doing household chores, tending to his fireplace, and even carrying firewood into the house from outside. The swelling had gone down. He was stronger, and he moved, talked, and expressed himself with new liveliness. The friend said that the once bedridden man had told him, "I feel I no longer have disease in my body."

The man continued to sleep grounded every night for the next five years until he died.

This remarkable turnaround is nothing more than Earth energy in action. It reveals the largely unknown fact that the ground represents the biggest and best natural antioxidant and anti-inflammatory that exists.

In this chapter, we will describe the healing connection between the Earth and physical inflammation. You'll get an idea how this connection has unlimited potential to reinfuse health and defuse pain among disconnected societies in which there is increasing sickness despite all the money poured into medical research and treatments.

But before we get back to the Earth and how it snuffs out inflammation, let's first look at what inflammation is (see the inset on opposite page).

Your immune system protects you against pathogens and facilitates the rebuilding of tissue at sites of injury or surgery. When a problem develops someplace, your body does the equivalent of calling 911. The alarm sounds. White blood cells and other specialized cells rush to the site—the first responders. The white blood cells constantly cruise throughout the tissues of your body, like police patrol cars, ever on the alert for viruses, bacteria, or other alien microorganisms, as well as damaged cells created by trauma or internal irritants. As weapons, some of the cells release a

---

What Is Inflammation?

Everyone is susceptible to inflammation—from high-performance athletes to non-performance couch potatoes. It's an equal opportunity hit man.

The word "inflammation" comes from the Latin *inflammatio,* meaning to set on fire. Inflammation is the complex biological response of the body to harmful stimuli, such as pathogens, damaged cells, or irritants. It is a protective attempt by the system to remove injurious or threatening agents as well as start the healing process for the affected tissue. In the absence of inflammation, wounds and infections would never heal and progressive destruction of the tissue would compromise survival.

---

shower of powerful free radicals (called an oxidative burst) that aid in the destruction of invading microorganisms and damaged tissue.

Free radicals have gotten a bad rap, and you will see why in a minute, but in reality they perform an essential service to the body. Simply put, they are positive-charged molecules (short of one or more electrons) that search for free electrons to become stable. You can call them electrophiles—electron lovers. Normally, these free radicals obtain their missing electrons by stripping electrons away from pathogens and damaged tissue. This activity kills the bad bugs you want out of your body and breaks down damaged cells for removal. As the remedial work winds down, excess free radicals produced during the immune response are neutralized by antioxidants or free electrons in the body.

This response is triggered whenever you have a disease or an injury. It is called the "inflammatory response." As a result, you may feel the familiar signs and symptoms of inflammation: swelling, redness, heat and pain, and, depending where the site is, decreased range of motion.

CHRONIC INFLAMMATION = ELECTRON DEFICIENCY

Inflammation comes in two forms: acute or chronic. The acute type takes place as an initial response of the body to harmful stimuli. It involves the mobilization of plasma (the yellow-colored liquid component of blood) and white blood cells from the blood into the injured tissue, as just described. That's okay. You want that to happen.

Then there is chronic (prolonged) inflammation. That you don't want. Chronic inflammation means a progressive shift in the type of activity going on at the site of inflammation. You get simultaneous destruction and healing of the tissue, but a harmful free-radical encroachment into healthy, surrounding territory. The destruction derby continues, and it can seriously harm you.

Free radicals obviously have starring roles in the immune response, but problems arise when the process fails to wind down completely after the job is done. The good guys become bad guys on a rampage, ripping up innocent, healthy cells. Think of security dogs that snag the burglar and then go after their owner. They continue attacking and oxidize healthy tissue. The immune system gears switch into overdrive, sending in more white blood cells that produce more free radicals. This activity is why free radicals have a bad rap and why scientists unanimously agree that free-radical activity is at the basis of chronic disease and the aging process, particularly accelerated aging and limited lifespan.

We believe that normal inflammation veers out of control because of lost contact with the Earth. People are suffering from an electron deficiency—not enough free electrons on hand to satisfy the lust of rampaging free radicals. They continue to attack the adjacent neighborhood of healthy tissue in an ever-expanding vicious cycle. The nonstop attack mode generates an autoimmune response manifesting as chronic inflammation. The immune system has run amok, attacking its owner—you.

We've simplified the scenario, but this is basically how it works. A destructive process unfolds that can continue silently and indefinitely even for dozens of years and lead to so many intractable modern diseases. Earlier we mentioned the new scientific term for this—inflamm-aging. Now you can see where it comes from.

INFLAMMATION AS A DISEASE-MAKER

The idea that chronic inflammation could be involved in disease began to gain serious attention a little over twenty-five years ago. At that time, two Australian researchers, Barry Marshall and Robin Warren, reported for the first time that stomach ulcers were not caused by stress or spicy food but by inflammation triggered during bacterial infection. This discovery earned the pair a Nobel Prize.

A similar kind of turning point in the road occurred recently in the field of cardiology. Back in the mid-1800s, the famous German pathologist Rudolph Virchow recognized that injured and inflamed arteries might be a source of heart attacks. His idea failed to gain traction during his time and faded away. Later, during most of the last half of the twentieth century, the cholesterol theory emerged, and since then lowering cholesterol has become a medical obsession and a multi-billion dollar business for pharmaceutical and food manufacturers. However, medical research has shown that half of all heart attacks and strokes occur among people with normal cholesterol levels. So during the 1980s, some cardiologists began to re-examine Virchow's ideas about inflammation.

A major breakthrough came in a series of important studies beginning in 2000. Evidence from a Women's Health Initiative study that monitored the status of 28,000 initially healthy postmenopausal women introduced a new cardiovascular risk factor into the spotlight: C-reactive protein (CRP), a biochemical substance indicating the presence of arterial inflammation. People with the highest level of CRP had five times the risk of developing cardiovascular disease and four times the risk of a heart attack or stroke compared to individuals with the lowest level. CRP, the researchers said, predicted risk in women who had none of the standard risk factors and was the best predictor among twelve risk factors studied, including cholesterol. Harvard cardiologist Paul Ridker, M.D., the lead researcher, said, "We have to think of heart disease as an inflammatory disease, just as we think of rheumatoid arthritis as an inflammatory disease."

Dr. Ridker estimated that approximately 25 percent of Americans have normal to low cholesterol, lulling them into complacency, but at the same time they have elevated CRP they don't know about. This means that millions of Americans are currently unaware they have an increased risk for future cardiovascular disease, heart attack, or stroke.

Think of low-grade inflammation as a silent, creeping fire, consuming arterial tissue. It leads to the weakening and eventual rupture of arterial plaques that directly trigger heart attacks and stroke. The CRP-inflammation link helps explain why so many heart attack and stroke victims have normal cholesterol levels.

Another example of a common disorder increasingly being seen as inflammation-related is diabetes. In type 1 diabetes, the kind that affects youngsters, the body's immune system attacks the pancreatic cells that make insulin. Insulin is the hormone responsible for controlling the blood sugar level and opening cell "doors" to sugar for use in energy production. Recent research also suggests that type 2 diabetes, the most common form of the disease and generally occurring in adulthood, begins with insulin resistance. This means that energy production stops responding properly to insulin. The reason for this, researchers believe, is an excess of inflammatory substances released from fatty tissue, particularly in the abdomen. Fat cells, once thought to be merely storage depots for energy and metabolically inert, are now known to be hotbeds of inflammation. This connection helps explain why obesity leads to diabetes. In addition, some studies suggest that eating certain foods may stoke more inflammation in the body and raise the risk of diabetes. They include foods high in sugar and other sweeteners, white flour products, trans fats, polyunsaturated vegetable oils, and processed meats.

It seems that hardly a day goes by without some new study pointing the finger at runaway inflammation as the core of some disease. Inflammatory diseases have become a global epidemic and include some of the most devastating disorders of our times. Table 6-1 lists just a few of them.

Along with the continuing flow of revelations regarding inflammation, researchers have also accumulated much evidence demonstrating that painful conditions are often the result of acute or chronic inflammation. One pain expert recently postulated that the origin of all pain is inflammation and the inflammatory response.

Many physicians and researchers wonder what has caused inflammation to become so dangerously commonplace. When asked what causes inflammation in the first place, Harvard's Dr. Ridker said this: "We are witnessing evolutionary biology in action—an adaptive response (inflammation) in the past is now maladaptive in our current modern environment."

The discovery of the relationship of grounding to inflammation suggests that the once adaptive response called inflammation has maybe gone sour because of an electron deficiency from loss of direct contact with the Earth.

TABLE 6-1. CONDITIONS RELATED TO CHRONIC INFLAMMATION

DISEASE	HEALTH EFFECTS
Allergies	Inflammatory messengers stimulate release of histamine, leading to allergic reactions.
Alzheimer's disease	Inflamed brain tissues develop plaque; chronic inflammation kills brain cells.
Amyotrophic lateral sclerosis (ALS)*	Damage to motor neurons causes the body to launch an overzealous inflammatory counterattack, killing the motor neurons.
Anemia	Inflammatory messengers attack red blood cell production.
Arthritis	Chronic inflammation destroys joint cartilage and inhibits the release of lubricating and cushioning fluid in the joints.
Asthma	Inflammation leads to blocking of the bronchial passages.
Autism	Brain inflammation is present in most autistic children.
Cancer	Inflammation contributes to free radicals, tumor growth, and inhibits the body's defense against abnormal cells.
Cardiovascular disease	Inflammation causes thick, unhealthy blood and arterial disease, leading to blockage and plaque and increased risk of dangerous clots in the blood vessels that feed the heart and brain; inflammation also damages heart valves.
Diabetes, types 1 & 2	Type 1 diabetes, inflammation induces the immune system to destroy pancreatic beta cells; type 2 diabetes, fat cells cause the release of inflammatory messengers, leading to insulin resistance.
Fibromyalgia	Inflammatory compounds present in the body at an elevated level.
Common intestinal disorders	Crohn's disease, irritable bowel, diverticulitis, and other intestinal problems involve inflammation that causes pain, interference with digestion and assimilation of nutrients, and damage to the sensitive lining of the digestive tract.
Kidney failure	Inflammation restricts circulation and damages kidney cells that filter blood.
Lupus	Inflammatory compounds spark an autoimmune attack.
Multiple sclerosis	Inflammatory compounds attack the nervous system.
Pain	Activation of pain receptors, transmission and modulation of pain signals, and hypersensitivity of nervous system are all one continuum of inflammation and the inflammatory response.
Pancreatitis	Inflammation induces pancreatic cell injury.
Psoriasis and eczema	Inflammation-based skin disorders.

*ALS is often called Lou Gehrig's disease

ENTER EARTHING: THE MISSING LINK

The land and seas of planet Earth are alive with an endless and constantly replenished supply of electrons. By making direct contact with the surface of the planet—the skin of our bodies touching the skin of the Earth—our conductive bodies naturally equalize with the Earth. Figuratively speaking, we refill the electron level in our tank that has become low.

How do we know that the body absorbs those electrons? There are a number of ways we know.

One is common sense. The Earth is negatively charged. It has an endless supply of negative-charged free electrons. Anytime you have two conductive objects and they make contact—such as your bare feet and the ground—electrons will flow from the place where they are abundant to the place where there are fewer of them. The electrical potential of the two objects will thus equalize. That's grounding. Similarly, when you stick a ground rod in the Earth, it allows the electrons to flow from the Earth via a wire into an object. It could be a refrigerator, the shielding around a cable TV system, or you. Your body is conductive like the fridge.

If you have a battlefront with positive-charged free radicals running amok inside your body, guess what's going to happen when you make contact with the Earth?

Big negative-charged Earth overwhelms little, positive-charged free radicals.

Science backs up the common sense. Science tells us that the body is one dynamic conductor of electrical impulses, or in the words of biophysicist James Oschman, "the living matrix." Cells contain an internal framework known as the cytoskeleton that connects all parts of the cell, from the nucleus to the outer membrane. This "scaffolding" includes molecules that conduct energy and information inside each cell and outward to the surrounding environment, and in the opposite direction, from the environment to the innermost parts of the cell and nucleus. Similarly, the surrounding environment, from your head to your toes, contains an extracellular network of conductive collagen and other proteins that are "hardwired" to cell membranes. Thus, the living matrix inside and outside cells provides a body-wide network for antioxidant electrons, a pathway hooking up all parts of the body, including the nervous system and all sensory receptors, with all parts of every cell, including the genome in every cell.

This pervasive system has extensions into every nook and cranny of the body and really represents, when you think about it, the largest organ system in the body. It is the "stuff" of all living structures.

When you think of yourself as an "antenna," as the French agronomist Matteo Tavera describes all living things (we discussed his ideas in Chapter 2), you can see how we fit neatly into a universal energy continuum. We, and the stars, are bathed in it.

Medical science utilizes the concept of the living matrix in a very practical and helpful way. Doctors use electrophysiological and biomedical instrumentation such as EKGs, EEGs (electroencepthalograms), and EMGs (electromyograms) as diagnostic tools to monitor the electrical activities of the heart, brain, and muscles. These devices follow certain conductive

Michael Jordan and the Living Matrix

Think of the living matrix as a kind of warp-speed communication network inside your body.

Nobel Prize winner Albert Szent-Györgyi, the Hungarian biochemist who first identified vitamin C and was among the first to apply theories of quantum physics to the understanding of cancer, was always a scientist ahead of his time. He laid out the vision of a high-speed communication system in the body—he called it "electronic biology"—back in 1941. He said, "Life is too rapid and subtle to be explained by slow-moving chemical reactions and nerve impulses. The proteins are the stage upon which the drama of life unfolds. The actors can be none other than small and highly mobile units such as electrons and protons."

To illustrate the blazing fast speed of communication within the living matrix, Dr. Oschman uses the analogy of Michael Jordan, one of professional basketball's greatest players. It is the last game and the last seconds of the basketball playoffs. The game is tied, and of course the ball comes to Jordan. In an instant he springs into mid-air and launches the ball toward the basket. As the buzzer sounds and the game is over, the ball drops through the hoop. Jordan's buzzer-beating shot wins the championship for his team. As the fans go wild, Jordan looks into the TV cameras, smiles, and shrugs his shoulders, as if to say, "Don't ask me how I did that!"

pathways existing between internal organs and the body skin surface, and vice versa. The readings from the interior follow pathways to the skin surface, where they are picked up by electrode patches and led to the measuring devices. Pacemakers, defibrillators, and electroacupuncture demonstrate how this conductivity works in reverse: from the skin to the tissues and organs inside the body.

Electrons are the smallest possible negative charges of electricity. It is well established that negative charges (electrons) are attracted to positive charges (free radicals). Connecting the body to the Earth automatically enables the conductive tissues of the body's living matrix to become charged with the Earth's free electrons. When this occurs, excess or residual immune response free radicals (which are positively charged) suddenly have, as the old song goes, the object of their affection—a readily available supply of free electrons to bond with and reduce their oxidative and inflammatory mode. They are neutralized, quenched, satiated, and satisfied. Kind of like giving kids the keys to the ice cream store or opening the blood bank to Dracula.

As a result, the addiction of immune system-produced free radicals to oxidize healthy tissue to obtain their fix of missing electrons naturally disappears. The rampage is naturally inhibited, and with it the underlying mechanism of chronic inflammation and autoimmune disease. The body naturally conducts, and becomes charged with, the Earth's free electrons; that is, it equalizes with and maintains the natural electrical potential of the Earth. The end result, our observations and research indicate, is that the reconnection prevents or reduces chronic inflammation and consistently speeds recovery from exhaustion, acute trauma, and minor injuries. You'll read how that plays out in the very dramatic stories we've collected in Part Four of the book.

Typically, there's a quick reduction in inflammation-related aches and pain. Some acute headaches can vanish within minutes. The intensity of chronic pains often lessens significantly in twenty to forty minutes.

The effect of Earthing on inflammation and pain was dramatically demonstrated in a series of case studies conducted with thermography during 2004 and 2005. Thermography, also known as infrared imaging, is a noninvasive clinical technique that analyzes the skin surface temperatures as a reflection of normal or abnormal human physiology. The technique utilizes sophisticated computerized technology to translate temperature data and produce an image that is then evaluated for signs of possible disease or injury. The procedure has been around for more than thirty years and featured in thousands of medical studies. Among other things, it is widely used to help diagnose breast cancer, diabetes, nervous system and metabolic disorders, injuries, headaches and pain syndromes, neck and back problems, and arterial disease.

William Amalu, D.C., president of the International Academy of Clinical Thermography, performed Earthing studies on twenty patients with a variety of complaints, including chronic myofascial pain syndrome, muscular strains, ligamentous sprains, peripheral neuropathies, carpal tunnel syndrome, inflammatory joint conditions, Lyme's disease, and chronic sinusitis. The subjects were either grounded with conductive electrode patches in his office or slept on grounded bed pads at home. The results showed, through dramatic pictures, a major and rapid impact on inflammation and pain. A picture is worth a thousand words, so please refer to the color images (Plates 1–7) on pages 69–74 showing some of these changes.

Some patients experienced improvement in just one session. Within two to four weeks (of two to three half-hour treatments weekly), up to 80 percent improvement occurred in the cases that were followed up (60 percent of cases were followed). With ongoing grounding over weeks and months, the patients continued to get relief, feel better, and in some cases, their symptoms vanished altogether.

"The moment your foot touches the Earth, or you connect to the Earth through a wire, your physiology changes," James Oschman says. "An immediate normalization begins. And an anti-inflammatory switch is turned on. People stay inflamed because they never connect with the Earth, the source of free electrons, which can neutralize the free radicals in the body that cause disease and cellular destruction."

THERMAL & PHOTOGRAPHIC IMAGES
OF THE EFFECTS OF EARTHING

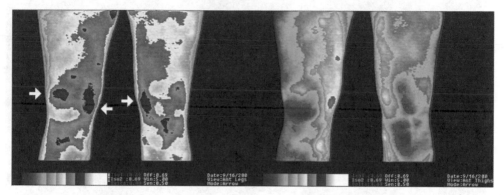

Plate 1. Inflammation as seen through infrared imaging. Thermal imaging cameras record tiny changes in the temperature of the skin to create a color-coded image map. Because tissue damage causes increased heat, abnormally hot areas indicate inflammation. The infrared photos shown here were taken only thirty minutes apart—before (left) and after grounding (right). They illustrate a rapid resolution of inflammation and help explain the impact of Earthing on chronic pain, stiffness, and a variety of symptoms.

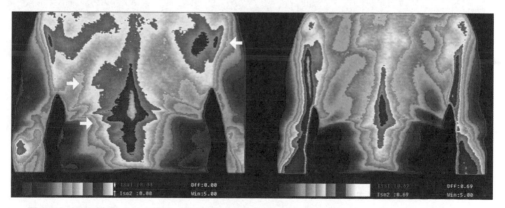

Plate 2. The patient here was an eighty-five-year-old male who complained of intense, left lower back pain and right shoulder pain that interfered with sleep, and waking stiff and sore. Prolonged medical treatment had achieved poor results. After two nights of sleeping grounded, he reported 50 percent less pain and 75 percent less stiffness and soreness when walking. Image (left) shows intense areas of inflammation and pain, denoted by arrows. Image (right), taken after second night, shows return to normal thermal symmetry. After four weeks, patient reported total resolution of back and shoulder pain with only occasional mild stiffness. "I have my life back," he said.

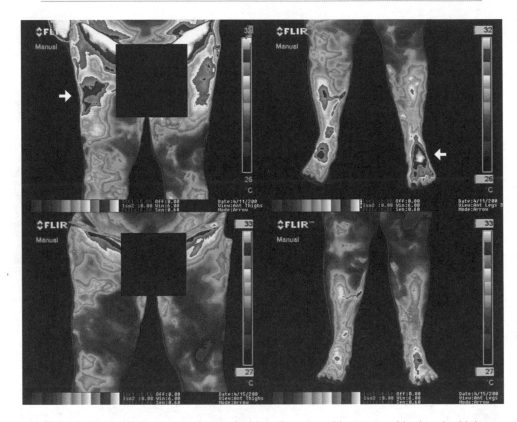

Plate 3. Infrared images are those of a sixty-five-year-old woman with chronic thigh, knee, and shin pain on the right leg, with ankle pain and swelling of the left foot. The patient complained of insomnia, nonrestful sleep, lack of sleep interfering with daily functioning, sleepiness during the day, pain interfering with sleep, leg achiness during sleep, and waking stiff and sore. She had been on prolonged medical treatment with poor results. After four nights of sleeping grounded on a conductive bed pad, the patient reported a 90 percent reduction in pain, a 50 percent improvement in restful sleep, and a 50 percent reduction in insomnia, sleepiness during the day, and waking stiff and sore. Steady continuous improvement was reported at a forty-day follow-up. Images (top) show the lower extremities taken before grounding. Arrows denote most significant areas of inflammation and correspond precisely with subject's areas of complaint. Images (bottom) were taken after four nights of sleeping grounded. Note the considerable reduction in inflammation and return toward a normal thermal pattern.

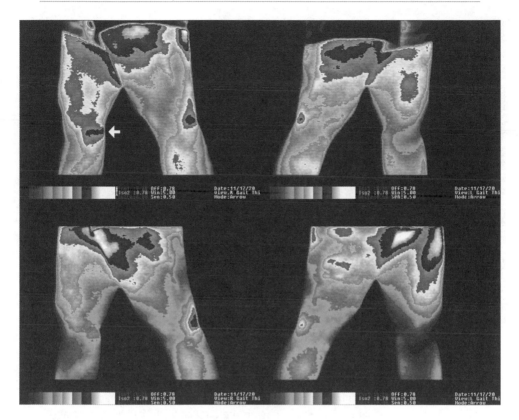

Plate 4. Infrared images are those of a thirty-three-year-old woman who had a gymnastics injury at age fifteen. The patient had a long history of chronic right knee pain, swelling, and instability, and was unable to stand for long periods. Simple actions, such as driving, increased the symptoms. She needed to sleep with a pillow between her knees to decrease the pain. On-and-off medical treatment and physical therapy over the years provided minimal relief. Images (top) were taken in walking position to show the inside of both knees. The arrow points to exact location of patient's pain and shows significant inflammation. Images (bottom) were taken thirty minutes after being grounded with an electrode patch. The patient reported a mild reduction in pain. Note significant reduction of inflammation in knee area. After six days of grounding, she reported a 50 percent reduction in pain and said that she could now stand for longer periods without pain and no longer needed a pillow between her legs when she slept. After four weeks of treatment, she felt good enough to play soccer and for the first time in fifteen years felt no instability and little pain. By twelve weeks, she said her pain had diminished by nearly 90 percent and with no swelling. For the first time in many years, she was able to waterski. Six months after initial treatment, she completed running a half-marathon.

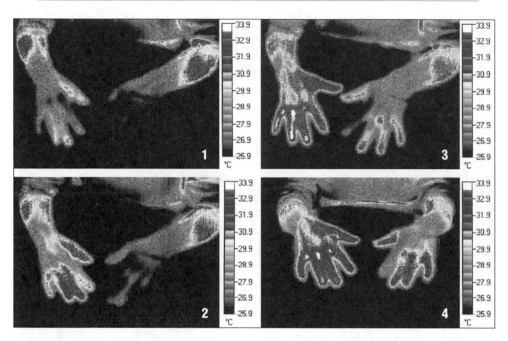

Plate 5. This set of infrared images relates to inflammation in the forearm tendons of a dental hygienist suffering from bilateral carpal tunnel syndrome. She was receiving three workers' compensation physical therapy treatments and three chiropractic treatments per week. Her symptoms included finger pain, coldness, and stiffness, and wrist pain. The forearm inflammation was reducing the circulation to her fingers. Image 1 shows the pre-treatment thermogram, revealing cool fingers and wrist due to poor circulation. Note the evidence of inflammation in the upper forearms. An Earthing electrode patch was placed on her left palm. Image 2 shows the delivery and distribution of blood to her right fingers after six minutes of Earthing. The fingers were beginning to get warmer. Image 3, after eleven minutes, shows continuing improvement of the circulation in the right fingers and wrist, and the beginning of improvement in her left fingers. Image 4 shows dramatic improvement on both sides after sixteen minutes. Note also the decrease in temperature (inflammation) in the upper forearms.

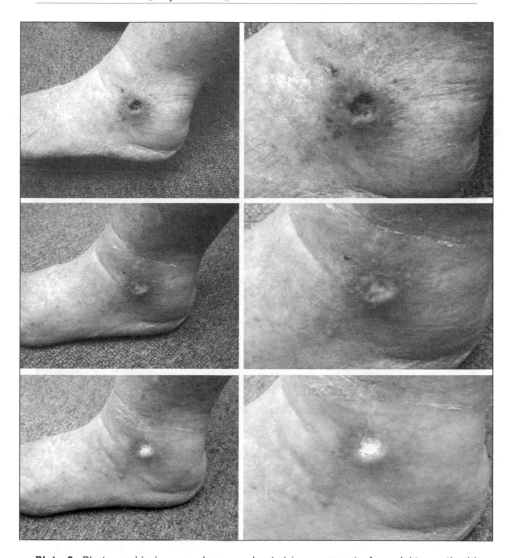

Plate 6. Photographic images show accelerated improvement of an eight-month-old nonhealing open wound suffered by an eighty-four-year-old woman. Right column pictures are close-ups of photos to the left. Top row shows the open wound and a pale-gray hue to the skin. Middle row photos, taken after one week, show marked level of healing and improvement in circulation, as indicated by the skin color. Bottom row, taken after two weeks, show the wound healed over and skin color looking dramatically healthier. Treatment consisted of a daily thirty-minute grounding session with an electrode patch while seated comfortably. The cause of the wound adjacent to the left ankle was a poorly fitted boot. A few hours after wearing the boot, a blister formed, and then developed into a resistant open wound. The patient had undergone various treatments at a specialized wound center with no results. Vascular imaging of her lower extremities

revealed poor circulation. When first seen, she had a mild limp and was in pain. After an initial thirty minutes of exposure to grounding, the patient reported a noticeable decrease in pain. After one week of daily grounding, she said her pain level was about 80 percent less. At that time, she showed no evidence of a limp. At the end of two weeks, she said she was completely pain free.

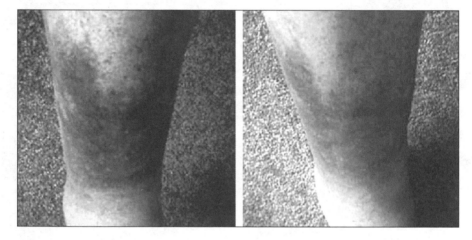

Plate 7. Effects of grounded sleep on a forty-seven-year-old male with diabetic neuropathy. Photo (left) is of the patient's lower right leg before treatment. After three nights of grounding with a conductive bed pad and electrode patches on both feet, the patient reported significant relief of pain and improved sleep. After seven nights, there was substantial reduction in redness and inflammation, indicating better circulation (right). The patient also reported great improvement in energy levels and an overall sense of "increased well-being."

CHAPTER 7

Connecting
the Dots

Gaetan Chevalier is a hard-nosed Southern California biophysicist and electrophysiologist, a scientist specializing in the body's electrical "wiring." In the summer of 2008, he conducted a study to investigate the impact of Earthing on a variety of physiological functions in the body. During preliminary work to test the design of the study, he invited a friend—a retired probation officer—to the laboratory to act as a "guinea pig." The subjects in the experiment were going to be grounded while sitting in a comfortable reclining chair, similar to one you may have in your living room. The friend sat down in the chair, and Clint Ober started chatting with him.

"A few minutes into the conversation, my friend mentioned that he had painful arthritis in his hands, something I hadn't known about," recalled Dr. Chevalier. "Clint then asked him to describe his current level of pain on a scale of 0 to 10, with 10 being unbearable pain.

"My friend described his level as 8 in the left and 9 in the right.

"Clint then placed an electrode patch on the palm of each hand and snapped on a wire connected to an outside ground rod. We continued to talk. After about a half hour, Clint asked my friend about the pain level now.

"A look of surprise came over my friend's face. He suddenly became aware that his pain level had dropped way down. He answered 2 on the left and 3 on the right, and then said, 'I have not experienced so little pain in my hands for a long time. This is amazing.'"

Dr. Chevalier described a similar experience with one of his yoga

75

instructors. She had severe arthritis in the thumbs, and doing something as simple as picking up an object—a cup, for instance—would often produce shooting pain up into the arm so bad that she dropped the object.

"She came to the laboratory and we grounded her for a half hour," he said. "When she left, she told us she didn't feel any pain. I see her every week at yoga class, and after several months she said that the pain in the thumbs never came back. She now walks on the beach for at least a half-hour every day and also sleeps grounded."

Observations like these have been commonplace right from the start of the pursuit of scientific validation for Earthing. The positive results in the early studies prompted deeper and more sophisticated investigations about how grounding affects the body and its complicated inner machinery. Now, a decade after the first experiment, ongoing research has started to put together the pieces of this amazing story into a multifaceted hypothesis with great implications for human health. In this chapter, we will present some of the most revealing and important findings to date.

THE NUTS AND BOLTS OF EARTHING

A study published in 2005 by electrical engineer Roger Applewhite confirmed two highly significant facts:

1. Electrons move from the Earth to the body and vice versa when the body is grounded. This effect is sufficient to maintain the body at the same negative-charge electrical potential as the Earth. We hypothesize that this flow of free electrons into the body is the mechanism by which inflammation is brought down.

2. Grounding powerfully reduces electromagnetic fields (EMFs) on the body.

It is hard to avoid electro-technical language to describe this important study that demonstrates some basic physics behind Earthing, and specifically that the human body is a natural conductor of the Earth's vibrant surface energy. We will do our best to keep things simple.

Mr. Applewhite is an expert in the design of electrostatic discharge systems for high-tech and electronic industries. His study, published in the journal *European Biology and Bioelectromagnetics,* involved a series of electrical measurements on the body of an individual grounded and ungrounded. Grounding was achieved by attaching conductive electrode patches to various places on the anatomy or by lying on a conductive bed sheet.

A voltage drop across an in-line resistor, measured with an oscilloscope, provided ample evidence of an exchange of electrons between the Earth and the body during grounding.

The electric potential (in volts) generated on the body by the EMFs at 60 Hz was recorded on both the ungrounded and grounded body using a specially designed high-impedance measurement system. Earthing, either with the patches or the bed sheet, reduced the immediate environmental electric potential by a factor of at least 70. Figure 7-1 below shows this knockdown effect graphically.

Thus, in one study, the Earth connection was shown to serve as a "source" of beneficial electrons and, at the same time, as a "shield" preventing environmental electric fields from creating disruptive electric potentials on the body.

EARTHING TRUMPS EMFS

In recent years, there has been much discussion in scientific circles and in the media about the possible health effects from exposure to man-made

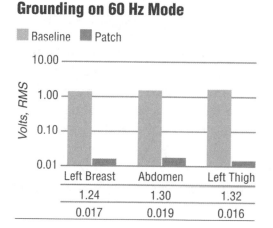

Effect of Conductive Patch Grounding on 60 Hz Mode

Baseline Patch

	Left Breast	Abdomen	Left Thigh
	1.24	1.30	1.32
	0.017	0.019	0.016

Figure 7-1.
The graph shows the huge difference in environmental electric field potential measured on the body at three sites—at baseline, that is, before grounding, and during grounding.

EMFs. Because of widespread interest in this issue, we would like to take a moment and attempt to shed additional light on the subject in relation to grounding.

All of us live immersed in an unseen sea of human-generated EMFs. They are everywhere—in our houses, workplaces, and outdoors—primarily produced by the electrical power grid. In North America, the grid produces EMFs vibrating at 60 Hz. Existing wires inside the walls produce EMFs even when appliances are not connected. The potential for interference in our bodies varies from person to person and in different locations, depending on the intensity of the fields. Within an ungrounded body, electrons and other charged particles react with the EMFs present in the immediate environment producing unnatural perturbations. When a person is grounded, the body is shielded from these perturbations by the Earth's electrons. An EMF has both an electric and a magnetic field, and the difference between the two and their effects on the body is explained in Appendix B, "The Physics of Earthing."

Some individuals are ultra-sensitive and can be severely affected. This "electrical hypersensitivity" cannot be explained by any known mechanisms, as the threshold for known interactions is at least fifty times higher than actual exposure levels. Nevertheless, we believe that such hypersensitivity is a real phenomenon and is directly related to a loss of natural grounding, the modern-day disconnect with the Earth. In Chapter 10, you will read two dramatic stories of individuals who suffered with debilitating electrical hypersensitivity and whose symptoms were improved by Earthing. To us, the ungrounded body "floats" in a tempest of random environmental energies and operates unstably, like a leaf in the wind.

The Applewhite study we just described showed that when the body is directly connected to the Earth, it is essentially shielded from electropollution. This finding confirms what is generally accepted in basic physics (see the inset "The Umbrella Effect of Earthing" on page 80) and also substantiates what we learned while doing the cortisol study described in Chapter 3. In that experiment, twelve subjects were grounded to the Earth during sleep. Their electrical field–induced body voltage, from exposure to common electrical wiring and cords near their beds, was measured before and after grounding.

What most people don't realize is that if you sleep with a lamp, clock, or radio next to your bed, the electric field from the wires will extend out to your body, even if the appliances are turned off. As measured by a volt-meter, in the bedrooms of the study subjects there was an average of about 3.3 volts pre-grounding. The level was significantly reduced, averaging 0.007 volts, when subjects slept on the grounded bed pads. The stark differences, and protective effect of grounding, are summarized in Table 7-1.

TABLE 7-1. ELECTRICAL FIELD-INDUCED VOLTAGE CREATED ON SUBJECTS' BODIES WHILE LYING IN THEIR OWN BEDS		
SUBJECTS	VOLTS BEFORE GROUNDING	VOLTS AFTER GROUNDING
1	3.94	0.003
2	1.47	0.001
3	2.70	0.004
4	1.20	0.002
5	2.70	0.005
6	1.67	0.005
7	5.95	0.008
8	3.94	0.008
9	3.75	0.010
10	2.30	0.009
11	5.98	0.020
12	3.64	0.006
AVG	3.27	0.007

Our conclusion is further supported by the findings of a team of researchers from the Imperial College in London and the University of Washington's Department of Environmental and Occupational Health Sciences. In a 2007 report, they said that measurements in an office setting showed that the electrical energies people are exposed to indoors for large periods of time escalate the risk of infection, stress, and degenerative diseases, and reduce oxygen uptake and activity levels. "The nature of

The Umbrella Effect of Earthing

The Applewhite study showed the protective effect of Earthing against environmental electrical fields. Another way to think of this is as an umbrella effect.

Let us look for a moment at the electrical properties of the Earth's surface and the way the Earth's energy influences our biology. In his classic *Lectures on Physics* from the early 1960s, Nobel Prize physicist Richard Feynman describes the Earth's subtle energies. The surface, as we have seen, has an abundance of electrons, which give it a negative electrical charge. If you are standing outside on a clear day, wearing shoes or standing on an insulating surface (like a wood or vinyl floor), there is an electrical charge of some 350 volts between the Earth and the top of your head (see drawing, left) if you are 5 feet 9 inches (1.75 m) tall. Keep in mind it is about zero volts at ground level.

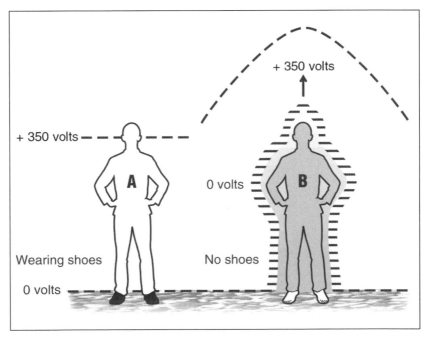

Figure 7-2. The umbrella effect of Earthing.

You might ask, "If there really is a voltage difference of 350 volts from head to toe why don't I get a shock when I go outside?"

The answer is that air is a relatively poor conductor and has virtually no electrical current flow. If you are standing outside in your bare feet (see drawing, right), you are Earthed; your whole body is in electrical contact with the Earth's surface. Your body is a relatively good conductor. Your skin and the Earth's surface make a continuous charged surface with the same electrical potential.

Also notice in the drawing on the right that the charged area is pushed up and away from your head if you are grounded. Any object in direct contact with the Earth—a person, a dog, a tree—creates this shielding effect. The object is essentially residing within the protective umbrella of Earth's natural electric field. This protective phenomenon also occurs inside your house or office, if you are connected to the Earth with an Earthing device like a bed pad.

the electromagnetic environments that most humans are now regularly exposed to has changed dramatically over the past century and often bears little resemblance to those created in Nature," they wrote. "In particular, the increased masking/shielding of individuals from beneficial types of natural electromagnetic phenomena, the presence of synthetic materials that can gain strong charge and increase exposures to inappropriate electric field levels and polarities have greatly altered the electromagnetic nature of the microenvironments many individuals usually occupy."

One of the factors contributing to the potential consequences of electropollution, they said, was the "failure to appropriately ground conductive objects (including humans)." For more technical reading on the possible risks of EMFs, lack of grounding, and living/working in high-risk settings, refer to Appendix B (section on "'The High Life'—A Voltage/Grounding/Health Connection?")

EARTHING PRODUCES UNIQUE ELECTRICAL FUNCTION IN BRAIN AND MUSCLES

In 2003, electrophysiologists Gaetan Chevalier and Kazuhito Mori at the California Institute for Human Science investigated the impact of Earthing on nervous system function. Fifty-eight healthy adults participated in the randomized, double-blind experiment involving a series of sophisticated brain and muscle measurements. In individual sessions, a conductive adhesive electrode patch was placed on the sole of each participant's foot while seated comfortably in a recliner. The patches were connected to a wire leading outside through a door. Half the participants were actually grounded, that is, the wire was connected to a ground rod, thus replicating the act of sitting or standing barefoot outside. The other participants were not grounded. They were similarly patched, but the wires were not connected outside to the rod. Individuals were then monitored, first for a half-hour pre-test baseline period and then immediately for another half hour when they were either grounded or "sham" grounded.

The sham group served as what researchers refer to as "controls." The purpose was to make sure the documented effects were real and not just due to people sitting and relaxing in a comfortable chair. The randomized experiment was double-blind, meaning that neither the participants nor the researchers knew which group was assigned to real or sham grounding. Blinded research is an important tool in many fields of research. Only after the data from the experiment have been recorded do the researchers learn who is who, enabling them to then analyze and compare the results.

EEGs record the electrical signals from your brain as measured on the scalp. Abnormal results may indicate the presence of epilepsy and seizures. EMGs detect the electrical voltage generated by muscle cells. In this study, EMG electrodes were placed on the big shoulder muscles on each side of the neck—the trapezius muscles, so named because of their diamond shape.

The EEG and EMG readings showed that grounding significantly influences the electrical activity of the brain and muscles, even within a mere half hour. In fact, dramatic changes were recorded almost instantly (within two seconds) of Earthing.

In the brain, there was an overall decrease in activity at all frequencies, with a crisp change showing on the left side—the one associated with thinking. Thus, Earthing appears to calm down the busy mind.

As far as the muscles were concerned, Earthing produced two intriguing results:

1. Participants with a high level of tension showed a decrease in muscle tension (on both sides). Individuals with little or no muscle tension

showed an increase in tension. The result suggests that grounding re-establishes a normal level of tension. The finding paralleled the effect of the earlier cortisol study in which a normalization of the stress-related cortisol level was seen.

2. The grounded subjects—but not the ungrounded ones—showed large and very slow oscillations (between twenty and forty seconds per oscillation, depending on the individual). This type of oscillation has never been seen before in physiology research.

Keep in mind that the body operates electrically, including your muscles. Nerve impulses instruct muscle fibers to contract. The contractions naturally generate electricity and small mechanical vibrations, both of which produce fluctuating frequencies of electrical potential at the surface of the skin. This is the electric "noise" that EMG measures. An oscillation (a slow vibration) means that the contractions generate electricity in a more rhythmic pattern. An analogy would be to compare people walking randomly in a crowd without any particular order versus a military unit marching in unison. The unit is more coherent than a random crowd. The influence of Earthing on muscles suggests more orderly and efficient activity.

The results of this study call for an experiment designed to determine whether greater electrical coherence translates to muscles being able to work longer and harder without fatigue. In Chapter 13, we present examples of grounded athletes describing enhanced performance, including one aging weightlifter who was able to substantially increase his lifting capacity. The implications for improved muscle function go far beyond athletes to the possibility that elderly individuals, at a time of life when they normally lose muscle strength, may achieve longer muscle "mileage" as a consequence of incorporating Earthing into their lifestyles. We believe the findings may represent a normal mode of muscle function not hitherto observed simply because no studies before have involved grounded subjects! Such precedence aside, the overall results provided additional proof of reduced stress and tension levels, and a shift in nervous system balance from a stress-stimulated sympathetic mode to a calmer parasympathetic mode. The study was published in a 2006 issue of the journal *European Biology and Bioelectromagnetics*.

EARTHING "ENERGIZES" MAJOR ACUPUNCTURE CHANNELS

When we walk barefooted, the front part of the sole (closest to the ball of the foot) comes in connection with the Earth. According to traditional Chinese medicine, this area includes a major acupuncture point known as kidney 1 (K1). The point is a major entryway for the absorption of Earth Qi—the Earth's energy—and connects further up in the body with the urinary bladder (UB) meridian. UB is an energy channel that reaches many of the most important organs and parts of the body, including the liver, diaphragm, heart, lungs, and brain, as well as a central meridian junction point in the back.

In a second phase of the electrophysiology study described a moment ago, Drs. Chevalier and Mori took the same fifty-eight participants and monitored them for nearly a half hour while ungrounded and then another half hour while grounded. Electrode patches were placed at the K1 point, thus simulating walking barefooted on the ground. (See Figure 7-3.)

The researchers wired up each participant and took detailed electrical measurements at more than two dozen meridian points on the body. They found that grounding generated readings indicative of reduced inflammation and energized internal organs. The results further supported earlier findings showing reduction of internal organ tension and inflammation, as well as increased parasympathetic activity in the nervous system.

Acupuncture Point

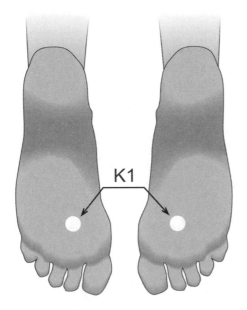

K1

Figure 7-3.
K1 acupuncture point.

This study suggests that "expressways" of electron transfer from the Earth through the body run through highly conductive water-control meridians (involving the kidneys and bladder) and the K1-UB "mainline" connecting many parts and organs of the body. The report was published in the journal *Subtle Energy and Energy Medicine* in 2007.

MORE EFFICIENT CARDIOVASCULAR, RESPIRATORY, NERVOUS SYSTEM FUNCTION

Reconnecting yourself to the Earth may not produce the same effect as jumpstarting a dead battery, but it does work surprisingly fast to re-energize fatigued bodies and reduce pain. Earthing usually generates a healing response that people feel after twenty to thirty minutes. Pain reduction can occur much faster.

In an attempt to clock the speed of Earthing, so to speak, a study was organized by Dr. Chevalier to measure different physiological values before, during, and after a forty-minute grounding session. Twenty-eight healthy men and women, ages eighteen to eighty, were used in the experiment. They were grounded with electrode patches applied to the soles of their feet and the palms of their hands. For comparison, measurements were also taken during a similar length session of sham grounding.

Actual grounding produced the following results:

- An immediate reduction (within a few seconds) of skin conductance, indicating rapid activation of the calming-mode parasympathetic nervous system. Skin conductance is a widely accepted measure of nervous system function. This result strengthens our understanding about stress reduction and improved sleep from grounding.

- An increased respiration rate and stabilization of blood oxygenation, as well as a slight rise in heart rate. These changes occurred about twenty minutes after grounding commenced and may suggest the start of a healing response necessitating an increase in oxygen. Signs of more efficient oxygen consumption during grounding continued, as was documented, for at least ten minutes after the cessation of grounding. This fascinating observation links Earthing and a healing response to metabolic activity. We hypothesize that this metabolic activity increase is the source of the healing response and that metabolic activity increases most where the body needs more repair, such as a site of injury or acute inflammation. Interestingly, immediately after ungrounding, blood oxygenation became erratic and respiration rate became even slightly higher. The reaction suggests that the body does not like being "unplugged" from the Earth.

The study, published in 2010 in the *Journal of Alternative and Complementary Medicine,* also showed that the more optimum measurements registered during forty minutes of Earthing shift back—in about ten to twenty minutes—to pre-grounding levels after the body is unplugged from the Earth.

POWER HEALING FROM TRAUMA: LESS INFLAMMATION, FASTER RECOVERY

You have undoubtedly experienced delayed onset muscle soreness after engaging in more physical activity than your body was used to. In the fitness and athletic world, this form of misery is called DOMS for short and is a well-known consequence of excessive, unfamiliar, or intensive exercise movements. Plain and simple: overdoing it.

There is no known treatment that reduces the recovery timeframe, but massage, hydrotherapy, and acupuncture have a reputation for reducing the pain. DOMS involves acute inflammation in the overtaxed muscles and develops in twenty-four to forty-eight hours. It can persist for well over ninety-six hours.

A study was set up using DOMS as a model to test the impact of Earthing on acute inflammation. Eight healthy males, ages twenty to twenty-three, were put through a similar routine of toe raises while carrying a barbell on their shoulders equal to a third of their body weight. The intense exercise was designed to create tissue injury and pronounced muscle soreness in the calves. In the experiment, each participant was exercised individually on a Monday morning and then monitored for the rest of the week while following a similar eating, sleeping, and living schedule in a hotel. For comparison, the group was divided in half. The men were either actually grounded or sham-grounded throughout the entire week—day and night.

The participants were objectively analyzed in a variety of ways, including through blood draw, MRI, MRS (magnetic resonance spectroscopy) of the injured tissue, and infrared thermal imaging. They were also tested daily for pain tolerance at the site of soreness—the calves. A blood pressure cuff was placed around their right gastrocnemius muscle (the big muscle at the back of the lower leg) and slowly inflated until the point of acute discomfort. The participants also provided subjective responses related to sleep, mood, and muscle soreness.

When inflammation occurs, white blood cells scurry into action. Their numbers increase. Among the ungrounded men, there was an expected, dramatic increase in white blood cells at the stage when DOMS is known to reach its peak and greater perception of pain (see Figure 7-4 on the following page). This result indicates a typical heightened inflammatory response. By comparison, the grounded group experienced a slight decrease in the white blood cell response, indicating almost no inflammation and, for the first time ever documented, a shorter recovery time. At twenty-four, forty-eight, and seventy-two hours after exercise, the white blood count differences between the two groups were 10, 17, and 18 percent.

The researchers looked at a total of forty-eight well-established markers of acute inflammation, DOMS, and pain. In thirty of these markers, a consistent pattern of differences emerged during the testing period.

The study, also published in 2010 in the *Journal of Alternative and Complementary Medicine,* was conducted under the supervision of Dick Brown, Ph.D., a well-known Oregon exercise physiologist and trainer of elite athletes.

"One big thing was the significant difference in the pain that these people felt," commented Dr. Brown. "The men who were grounded not only had a subjective feeling of less pain, but they could also take more pressure applied to their calves with the blood pressure cuffs. Their calves seemed to be less sore.

"Another big thing was the significant differences in the white blood cells and certain compounds in the body. These outcomes clearly invite more investigation, which we plan with a larger subject population.

Nighttime Pain Scale

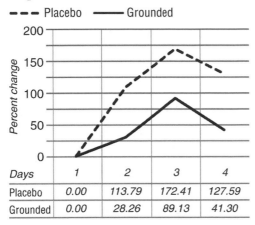

Days	1	2	3	4
Placebo	0.00	113.79	172.41	127.59
Grounded	0.00	28.26	89.13	41.30

Figure 7-4.
Delayed muscle onset soreness study.

Ungrounded subjects consistently, at every measurement taken, expressed the perception of greater pain. The differences ranged from 61 to 126 percent (top graph). Related to this finding was evidence of a subdued white blood cell response, indicating an Earthed body experiences less inflammation (bottom graph).

White Blood Cells

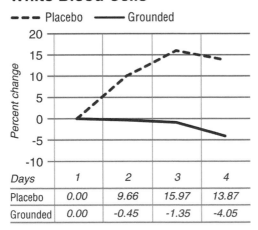

Days	1	2	3	4
Placebo	0.00	9.66	15.97	13.87
Grounded	0.00	-0.45	-1.35	-4.05

"I now tell the athletes I train to make every effort to ground themselves. They willingly do so because they have a sense that something is working. They say they have less pain, and that allows them to train more consistently and recover faster. That's a big deal because consistent training is so important to success.

"I personally experienced the benefit of grounding when I had a right knee replacement in 2009. I needed it after years of being physically active at a fairly high level. This is my second knee replacement surgery. The first was ten years ago. Subjectively, I felt I was improving a little bit faster. But five weeks after the operation, when I went to the surgeon for a checkup, he looked at my leg and looked at my movement and said, 'At five weeks, you are where most people are at three months.' He was speaking in terms of movement, wound healing, and swelling. I obviously attribute that partly to my knowledge of rehabbing, but the grounding certainly didn't hurt, and I honestly believe it helped. It had a positive effect.

"I sleep grounded, and I also use grounded electrode patches locally. Before surgery, I noticed that when I put the patches on the area of the knee that was hurting, it definitely reduced the pain compared to when I didn't have the patches on. I needed surgery for about a year but kept putting it off because I had things to do. And so at night, my leg got really painful. So I slept on the grounded sheet and slept better, and further knocked the pain down with the patches."

The careful process of scientific experimentation in the Brown study shows that inflammation is reduced and documents why Earthing has caught on big time in the sports world, where living with inflammation and injury is a way of life. Simply put: the body is different—and heals much faster—when connected to the Earth. Earthing = Power Healing.

REDUCED RISK OF METABOLIC SYNDROME

Preliminary results from an ongoing animal study revealed significant improvements from Earthing in several biochemical factors associated with metabolic syndrome in humans, a widespread—and rapidly growing—precursor to obesity, diabetes, and cardiovascular disease. The substances monitored were alkaline phosphatase (an enzyme), triglycerides, blood sugar, and C-reactive protein (a widely used indicator of chronic inflammation discussed in the previous chapter).

The values of these substances were considerably lower in grounded animals, suggesting they have less risk for metabolic syndrome. Just as in the DOMS study, there were also fewer white blood cells measured.

In this experiment, two healthy groups of thirty rats each were used. One group was housed in cages fitted with grounded mats. The control animals lived in similar, but ungrounded, cages. Blood samples were taken every month for six months and analyzed. Continued grounding resulted in progressive improvements. For this reason, the study was extended beyond the first six months of data collection. Final results are expected in mid-2010.

The preliminary results of this animal study tie in neatly with the increase in metabolic activity documented in the earlier experiment with human subjects where a relationship between Earthing and a more efficient cardiovascular, respiratory, and nervous system function was observed. It makes sense that an increase in metabolic activity results in a lower risk of developing metabolic syndrome.

Although we don't have the final conclusion yet from this study, we believe that preliminary results, along with other observations over the years, permit the suggestion—if nothing more at this time—that living in an ungrounded state may create another important cause of metabolic syndrome. One has only to look at today's youth, who generally consume large amounts of inferior quality convenience food and drinks high in

Earthing and Weight Loss? Maybe!

Abdominal obesity is one of the important factors characterizing metabolic syndrome. While abdominal obesity was not measured during the rat study above, the animals were weighed in at the first pre-test day and then again at each monthly blood collection time. The random difference in average weight between the two groups of "middle-aged" female rats at the beginning of the study was only 1.2 percent (the ungrounded rodents happened to be insignificantly heavier at the start than the grounded animals) and then grew steadily each month to reach 3.7 percent after six months, the last date that we have received data in this ongoing study.

What the numbers mean is that the ungrounded group added an extra 2.6 percent in weight after six months. Both groups were fed the same type and quantity of food. While the difference seems like a trifling amount, it translates to an extra five pounds for a person weighing 200 pounds. At that rate, by mid-2010, when the study will end, the difference in weight could grow to 7.8 percent, the equivalent of an extra sixteen pounds for a 200-pound person.

The results, along with the biochemical differences cited in the study, suggest that the grounded rats function at a higher metabolic efficiency than ungrounded animals.

Do these preliminary results infer that Earthing can generate weight loss in humans? We can't say. The prospect is certainly tantalizing. Imagine losing weight without doing anything. A dieter's dream.

sweeteners and calories, who are increasingly sedentary, and who wear insulated running shoes from morning to night. For young people as well as for adults, the unholy trinity for metabolic syndrome, and the serious disorders it gives rise to, may thus be poor diet, lack of exercise, and lack of grounding. It is something to think about.

According to the American Heart Association, metabolic syndrome is characterized by a group of metabolic risks that include the following:

- Excessive fat tissue in and around the abdomen.

- Blood fat disorders—high triglycerides, low "healthy" HDL cholesterol, and high "harmful" LDL cholesterol—that contribute to plaque buildups in arterial walls.

- Elevated blood pressure.

- Insulin resistance or glucose intolerance—conditions that interfere with the body's ability to properly use insulin or blood sugar.

- A tendency to form clots in the blood.

- A pro-inflammatory state in the body, that is, the presence of chemical substances associated with inflammation (such as elevated CRP).

THE EARTHING HYPOTHESES

The studies we have been describing have uncovered a simple but powerful fact: people who are grounded function better than they do ungrounded. They are, in fact, different. Based on the research, two scientists who have extensively studied and written about Earthing have made a number of intriguing hypotheses. They are James Oschman, Ph.D., and electrophysiologist Gaetan Chevalier, Ph.D.

The following is a summary of these ideas.

Living Longer and Better

Anti-aging medicine involves the search for factors that can restore and maintain adequate energy resources and the circulation of vital energy throughout the body. This quest has been going on with humans throughout history. It's nothing new.

Our research clearly shows that grounding has a powerful influence on the delicate balance between health and illness, and looming behind that, the prospect of living longer and better. This anti-aging prospect is clearly one of Earthing's most attractive aspects.

The dominant theory of aging—the concept of free-radical oxidative damage to the body—was first proposed by Denham Harman, M.D., of the University of Nebraska in 1956. The idea here is that aging results from the cumulative damage to the body produced by free radicals. These molecules can damage DNA, leading to mutations and disease. They are formed by metabolic processes in mitochondria, the "power plants" inside cells, and can gradually harm mitochondrial functioning and energy production throughout the body. They cause cross-linking of proteins, chemical reactions that interfere with normal enzyme activity. This is what causes skin to wrinkle for example. There is no way to prevent the formation of free radicals, because every breath we take and every morsel of food we eat feeds the natural mitochondrial production of energy and free radicals as a byproduct. Because of the constant threat of free radicals, we are encouraged to eat foods rich in antioxidants.

The living matrix, as one of its main biological functions, is set up to protect tissues from free-radical damage. It represents a natural, built-in antioxidant defense system. The matrix is all-pervasive, reaching into every corner of the body. If your matrix functions properly, and if you are connected to the Earth, any free radical formed anywhere in your body will be neutralized by mobile electrons from the Earth. This idea alone should motivate anyone to connect with the Earth as much as possible, day and night.

By understanding that the living matrix is a conductive fabric extending throughout the body, and that grounding connects this system to the Earth and an infinite source of free electrons, one can see that Earthing could prove to have far-reaching anti-aging, antioxidant, and anti-inflamm-aging effects. Long-term, controlled animal studies will enable us to verify or refute this profound hypothesis.

Research done in Germany has described the matrix in terms of a systemic reservoir of charges designed to maintain electrical balance and supply electrons in times of normal inflammatory need. Earthing provides recharging and keeps the reservoir full. Disconnection from the Earth dries up the reservoir.

A New Definition of "Normal" Immune Response

A common deficiency of electrons in the ungrounded body appears to distort and weaken the function of the immune system. But it can be readily restored to normal functioning by Earthing. The research suggests that Earthing may, in fact, create a whole new definition of what is a "normal" immune response.

As explained in Chapters 2 and 6, the inflammatory basis of disease has become a major focus of biomedical research. It is becoming widely accepted that chronic inflammation and chronic diseases, including so-called diseases of aging, are closely related. The classical inflammatory response may actually be an abnormal condition caused by separation from the Earth's readily available bank of free electrons. When the body is connected to the Earth, the classical signs and symptoms of inflammation are greatly reduced or absent, among them pain.

Promotes Healing of Injuries

The body forms an "inflammatory barricade" around sites of injury, where the immune system focuses on elimination of pathogens and damaged tissue. Free radicals involved in this process can spread from these sites and attack nearby healthy tissue, leading to chronic inflammation.

Earthing research gives the impression that free electrons can penetrate the barricade and thereby neutralize free radicals that have accumulated in pockets of inflammation. This ability appears to be a factor in accelerated healing.

A New Definition of "Normal" Physiology

When the body is connected to the Earth, a variety of beneficial physiological changes take place instantly. The studies that utilized a conductive patch placed on the bottoms of the feet and the palms of the hands made it possible to record the precise instant of connection to the Earth and document the sharp differences in various physiological parameters before and after grounding.

As scientific investigations continue, we expect to see countless more changes. The changes suggest that normal physiology may require a whole new set of ranges and definitions.

Restoring Your Internal Electrical Stability

The body evolved utilizing Earth's electrical energy (ground) to maintain its internal electrical stability for the normal functioning of all self-regulating and self-healing systems. The modern way of life prevents contact with the Earth most of the time, creating electrical instability. This lack of stability results in body system dysfunctions that lead to inflammation, inflamm-aging, disease, and aggravation of existing disorders.

The Earth serves the human body as a source of energy similar to a power line feeding electrical energy into electrical equipment and appliances. It is widely accepted that equipment will not function well without a ground. We recently rented a very sophisticated oscilloscope for graphing electrical signals with the most advanced technology, and yet when improperly grounded, the equipment did not function well. There was a need for a stable reference point. The Earth also plays that role for living beings, including human beings. To read more technical information about the electrical effects produced by grounding, refer to Appendices A and B.

Resetting Your Biological "Clocks"

Biological clock systems are found not only in humans and mammals, but in lower organisms as well, such as fish and insects. They are linked to survival. Although the human body packs several biological clocks (called peripheral clocks), researchers have found they are all under the control of a master clock located in the head, more precisely in the suprachiasmatic nucleus, a pair of distinct groups of cells in the hypothalamus.

One of the most important hypothalamic functions is to connect the nervous system to the endocrine system via the pituitary gland, the master gland of the body. Through hormonal secretions, it governs a multiplicity of activities affecting all body systems. Another function of the hypothalamus is to control the secretion of adrenocorticotropic hormone from the anterior pituitary gland, which in turn stimulates the secretion by the adrenal cortex of cortisol (the stress hormone). This system is so important for understanding the stress response that it is known as the hypothalamic–pituitary–adrenal axis.

The master biological clock receives its clues about prevailing light conditions from specialized cells in the retina. Signals about light conditions travel from the hypothalamus to the pineal gland, which controls the secretion of melatonin. Melatonin is secreted only in conditions of darkness.

The biological clocks control virtually all body system functions, including, of course, the wake-sleep circadian cycle.

From our research, we believe that not only light conditions but Earth's energy as well coordinates the various biological clocks regulating hormone flow in the body. The slow and gentle rhythms of the Earth's energy field are essential for maintaining these clocks. One example we have discussed is the day/night cortisol rhythm that is normalized when sleep is improved through grounding. Another example is the secretion of melatonin, which happens at night. Melatonin is widely known as a sleep-promoting factor. Since we have seen in our earlier studies that grounded people sleep better, we hypothesize that the rhythm of this hormone is also normalized when sleeping grounded. Any such normalization effect is important because melatonin is a powerful antioxidant, a major protector of the brain by preventing loss of brain cells by self-inflicted death. Given that a variety of neurodegenerative diseases, such as Alzheimer's disease, Parkinsonism, and amyotrophic lateral sclerosis (Lou Gehrig's disease), have a free-radical component, it is assumed that melatonin may be useful in forestalling the consequences of these debilitating conditions and improving the psychological health of these patients. Researchers are postulating also that melatonin has several major functions that probably help to protect against psychiatric illnesses.

At any point on the surface of the planet, the Earth's energy potential fluctuates according to the position of the sun and the moon, creating cycles such as the circadian cycle. This understanding helps to explain how passengers, after long flights across many time zones, can reset their internal clocks to "local time," so to speak, and quickly reduce the effect of jet lag by going barefoot or grounding themselves after arriving at their destination.

Our overall working hypothesis is that grounding leads to a much greater physiological stability because the diverse bodily rhythms are coordinated not only with the light/dark cycle, but with all the natural rhythms of the environment.

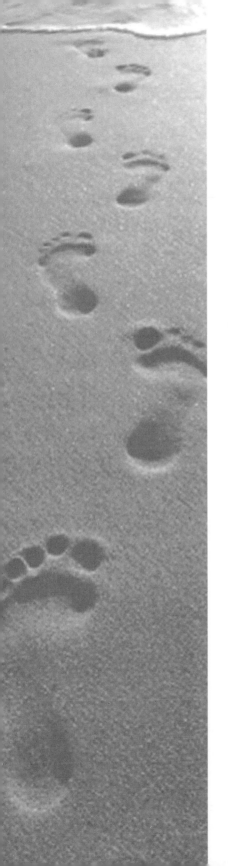

PART FOUR

The Earthing
Chronicles

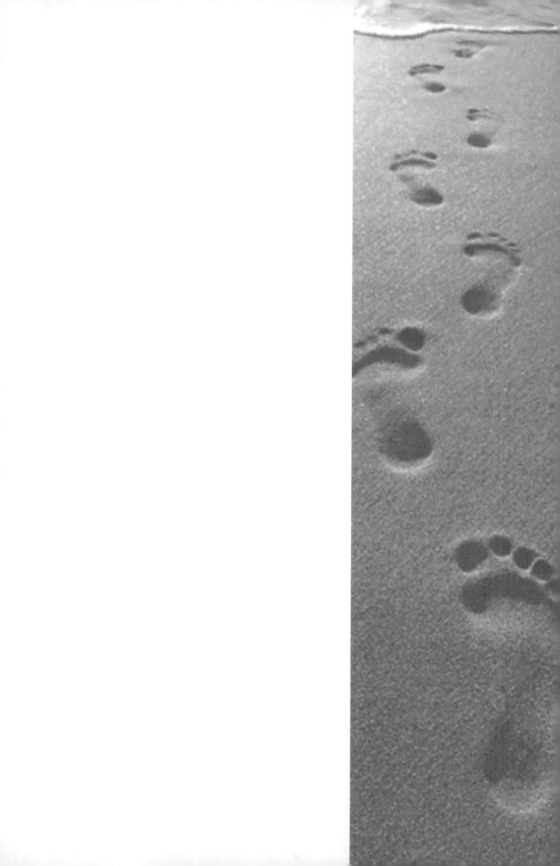

CHAPTER 8

Earthing 101: How to Connect

We have told countless people to walk barefoot in their backyards, on the beach, in a grassy park, on concrete or open ground, or any place outside wherever comfortable (and of course, where the surface is safe to walk on), and when the weather allows.

The feedback is inevitably one of surprise and delight:

"I feel so much better."

"I don't know what it is, but something changed for the better."

Everybody knows that walking is a healthy way to get physical activity. During the day it's also a good way to get vitamin D. You get sunshine's vitamin D from above, *plus* the anti-inflammatory energy from the Earth below.

Physical activity. Vitamin D. Earth energy. It's a trifecta!

Of course, Earth's energy is there for your taking any time, day and night. It's free. Nobody has to pump it into your body like gasoline in a car. It's not a pill. It's not a potion. It's not an ointment. It's just something in the ground, on the ground, and from the ground right there beneath your feet. It's always been there and always will. You can have as much of it as you want. No limit.

Everybody talks about "green energy" these days. This is Earth energy —both the original and ultimate form of green energy for your body and well-being.

Remember that the sole of the foot has more nerve endings, inch for inch, than any other part of your body. That's also where the acupuncture K1 point is located, with connections running up and through the body. So think of the soles of your bare feet as a prime contact point gathering in the free electrons and natural energies from the Earth.

Here's another feature of the sole: it is endowed with more sweat glands than any place else on your anatomy and perspires more than any part of the body, except your head and hands. Nature is the ultimate designer. The moisture helps conduct the electron flow from the ground up into your bioelectrical body. Nylons and cotton socks are okay. Moisture will penetrate them. But barefoot is best.

BAREFOOTING OPPORTUNITIES

Besides walking barefoot, you can, of course, ground yourself by sitting on the Earth or on a chair with your feet planted on the ground, while reading a book, listening to music, or just plain relaxing. For people with foot issues or tender feet, we recommend sitting in a comfortable chair with your bare feet placed directly on the Earth.

To make the Earthing experience most effective, dampen the soil or grass for added conductivity. Leave your feet squarely on the Earth and sit there for thirty or forty minutes. Actually, when any part of your body— your hands, forearms, legs, for example—makes contact with the ground, you are receiving the energy from below.

If you have the opportunity, connect with the Earth two or three times a day. The more time you put in, the more you benefit. The more compromised your health is, the more often and longer we recommend that you do this. But even in a half hour or so, you will have a remarkable shift. We have already measured some important physiological improvements within a half hour to forty minutes, and many more will come to light with continued research.

If you can't do these things outside, a concrete basement floor is a good venue, if you have one in your house. Dampen the area around your feet as well to enhance conductivity. Concrete, by the way, is a conductive substance, made from water and minerals. It sits on the Earth and retains moisture. So the free electrons will pass through just as they will if you are sitting or standing on grass or open ground. If the concrete is painted or sealed, there may not be any conductivity. Asphalt is made from petrochemicals and is not conductive. So don't expect any benefits from walking on painted or carpeted concrete or asphalt. The same goes for a wood or vinyl surface.

Water-wise, wading or swimming in the ocean is a great recreational form of grounding. Salt water, rich in minerals, is highly conductive, and actually several hundred times more so than freshwater. Conductivity depends on the concentration of minerals in the water. So lake water is much less conductive than salt water. And pool water is likely less than that. A plastic kiddie pool would not be conductive because the plastic would insulate the water from ground contact.

The amazing thing about Earthing is that it is so simple and fundamental. James Oschman, the energy-medicine expert, reports on new technologies emerging every day and is often asked to examine them and explain how they work. "What is most profound about Earthing," he says, "is the element of simplicity. I once attended a meeting on the East Coast, and one of my colleagues came in from the West Coast. She had a bad case of jet lag. I told her to take her shoes and socks off and step outside on the grass for fifteen minutes. When she came back in, she was completely transformed. Her jet lag was gone. That is how fast grounding works. Anyone can try it. If you don't feel well, for whatever reason, just make barefoot contact with the Earth for a few minutes and see what happens. Of course, if you have a medical problem, you should see a doctor. But for ordinary aches and pains, digestive or respiratory problems, or sore muscles, there is nothing that comes close to grounding for quick relief. You can literally feel the pain begin to drain from your body the instant you touch the Earth."

For many people, it may not be practical or possible to connect barefoot or bare-skinned with the Earth. The weather may be lousy and the prospect of freezing one's tootsies is hardly appealing. Or if the weather is good, contemporary living is so fast-paced that a meaningful hookup with the Earth may not be possible. There may not be time for a "barefoot break" during the daily routine. Or the thought of going barefoot may just not be appealing.

You would be surprised to know, however, that there is something of a "barefoot movement" going on. A lot of people are thumbing their noses at convention and going unshod for significant portions of their daily life.

A 2009 article in the Toronto *Globe and Mail* says that shoelessness is catching on—big time. Jennifer Yang wrote that "the Facebook fan page 'Being Barefoot' boasts more than two million fans, and . . . is one of the fastest-growing pages on the social networking site, according to a trend-tracking website, Inside Facebook. Across the Internet the 'barefoot lifestyle' is booming, with adherents turning to websites such as the Society for Barefoot Living (www.barefooters.org), with more than 1,200 members."

As far as the winter is concerned, one barefooter whom Ms. Yang interviewed was a sixty-four-year-old retired autoworker from southern (that's an important climate distinction in Canada) Ontario who has been mostly shoeless for fifteen years. "He even pads around barefoot during the winter," she wrote, "though he draws the line at temperatures below minus 18." That's zero Fahrenheit, and at that point, "he reluctantly slips on flip-flops." He, like most of the other shoeless converts, says that shoelessness feels more natural and healthier.

Comfort and naturalness aside, what's interesting about the current barefoot boom is that these unshod folks are picking up healing energy from the Earth and they very likely don't know it.

In the past, we all walked, sat, stood, and slept directly on the Earth. It was not a hardship. It was a way of life. Now, nobody in our industrialized society except Scouts, soldiers, backpackers, and backyard pajama-partyers sleep on the ground anymore.

One way to address the personal energy deficit that clearly exists as a result of our physical separation from Earth is to develop methods capable of being used while sleeping and sitting for prolonged periods.

BAREFOOT SUBSTITUTES

During more than ten years of scientific research and experimentation, Clint Ober used medical electrode patches and developed various prototypical bed pads, sheet sets, floor and desk pads, and sheet-like sleeping bags meant for travel and athletes. He even created a cushiony pad for indoor pets.

These devices, designed primarily for research, hold promise as barefoot "substitutes" that can provide inside connectivity to the Earth outside. They are connected by a wire to a ground rod placed directly in the Earth or plugged into the ground port of a grounded electrical outlet. They can be utilized during sleep, work, and even while watching TV. For information on development and availability of these Earthing devices, refer to Appendix C, "Resources."

All such paraphernalia do nothing restorative by themselves unless they are connected to the Earth. They are simply conductors of the Earth's natural energy to the body when you are indoors or unable to go barefoot. The Earth does the magic. They replicate standing barefoot or lying directly on the Earth. We like to think of them as extension cords connecting you to the Earth. With any of them, your body is immediately brought to the same electrical potential as the Earth.

Earthing Shoes

This is not a new principle. Specially grounded shoes are used in the electrostatic discharge industry to prevent buildup of static electricity in the body that could damage delicate electronic parts and chips.

By comparison, Earthing footwear will be designed with conductive inserts for everyday use, including popular flip-flops and sandals, allowing people to avoid the barefoot hazards of walking on surfaces containing pesticides, debris, and animal waste. When out and about, they will receive the health benefit of walking, plus a dose of healing free electrons. This concept gives "power walking" a new meaning.

In northern zones during the winter, conductive shoes and boots would give people an opportunity for outdoor Earthing under conditions when few people will venture forth barefooted.

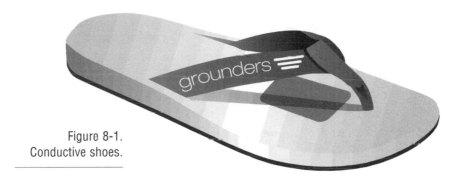

Figure 8-1.
Conductive shoes.

Universal Earthing Pads

Universal chair/desk/mouse/bed/floor mats and pads can be used inter-changeably to fit any setting. A pad placed on a desktop conducts through your forearms or wrists, on the floor through your feet, and on your chair through your butt. And on the bed through any part of your body that makes contact with it. Normal perspiration through layers of clothes, such as a dress, pants, socks, or long sleeves, permits varying degrees of con-ductivity. The pad utilizes a metallic fiber mesh and conductors coupled to a wire connected to a grounded outlet in the wall or to an outside ground rod.

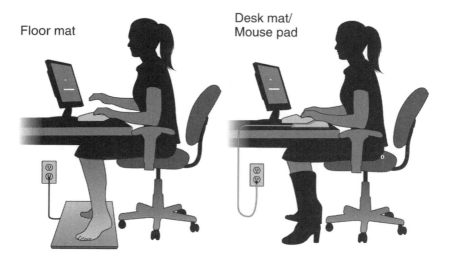

Figure 8-2. Universal pads.

Earthing Sheets

One major and highly practical application of Earthing has involved peo-ple sleeping or resting on a conductive half or full sheet connected to the Earth. Looking to the future, it is our expectation that the mattress and bedding industry will see the obvious appeal of incorporating Earthing technology. We expect the industry to step up with a wide array of ground-ing products. Figure 8-3 demonstrates the concept, using the example of a conductive half-sheet.

Contact with the Earth during the third of our lives we spend sleeping yields great benefits, as we have discussed in the previous chapters. The research to date indicates that Earthing during sleep is the ideal way of reducing oxidative stress and inflammation throughout the body. Sleep is the time when the body rests and recovers from the stresses of daily activities. If we do not sleep well, the recovery process works only partially, making us susceptible to a wide variety of stress-related problems. As these problems worsen, they can further interfere with our sleep, making the situation even worse.

Earthing sheets

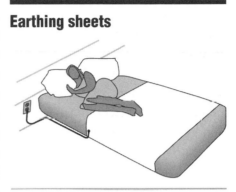

Figure 8-3. Sleeping on conductive sheet or half sheet.

This cycle of discomfort, stress, and insomnia can be readily reversed and improved in the majority of cases by sleeping grounded. Some people who have grounded themselves at night have thrown out their sleeping aids.

One woman, after sleeping grounded, described her experience thusly: "It's as if there's a big bulge in the wire carrying the Earth itself full of flowers, green grass, and animals, right into my bed. I feel as if I am lying there surrounded by Nature."

Earthing Mattress

An Earthing mattress is a natural sleep and health aid. Think of it as an "Earthing bed." People buy a new mattress every seven or eight years. So why not buy one with a grid of conductive material built into the mattress fabric? The addition represents an extremely low-cost upgrade to standard mattresses. In addition to comfort and rest, Earthing mattresses would improve health and lessen pain—as you sleep! Just lie down, go to sleep, get a treatment, and wake up feeling better and with more energy.

Like the conductive sheets and other barefoot substitutes, such a mattress would be connected to a ground rod outside or through a properly grounded outlet in the bedroom. A simple conductive sheet, without a snap for a wire connection, would be used over the mattress so that it makes contact with the conductive fabric in the mattress. Since mattresses are home delivered from the stores where they are purchased, it would

Earthing bed

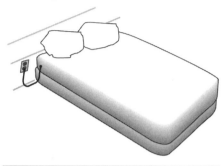

Figure 8-4. The "Earthing bed."

be simple for the deliverymen to not only set up the mattress in the home but also to check for proper grounding and connect it up. We expect the Earthing bed to be the next big thing in the mattress industry. This should, in fact, be the new standard for mattresses.

Earthing Recovery Bags

Recovery bag

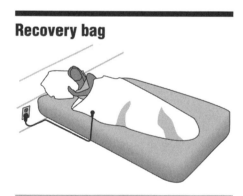

Figure 8-5. The recovery bag for athletes and travelers.

This conductive bag was created specially for Tour de France cycling teams and other athletes for the purpose of accelerating recovery from extreme physical activity. Users slip between the top and bottom sheet, as they would a sleeping bag, while resting or sleeping. This device can be rolled up and stuffed in a small cloth tote. It has become very popular with travelers and many athletes. We discuss more on the remarkable effect of grounding athletes in Chapter 13.

Electrode Patches and Body Bands

Many of our scientific experiments have utilized electrode patches similar to the kind used by doctors for EKG, EEG, and other electrical activity diagnostics. The conductive patches can be attached near an injury or wound or area of acute pain to accelerate the healing process and reduce local inflammation and discomfort. Athletes have found them to be especially effective against common injuries and strains.

Conductive patches

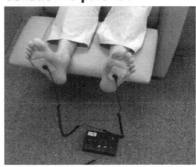

Figure 8-6. Electrode patches.

After experiencing quick pain relief, several participants in early grounding studies referred to the patches as "magic pain patches."

Some individuals, seeking concentrated relief for local pain (for example, in the arm, shoulder, or knee), have wrapped their grounded sheets or bed pads around the affected area. This is similar to using a grounded electrode patch and sticking it on or near a wound or a site of pain.

Body and knee bands

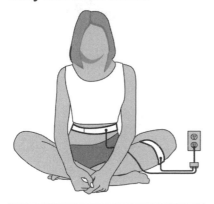

Figure 8-7. Velcro body bands.

We regard the grounded electrode patches as more of a research tool or a potential clinical aid that physicians may consider in the treatment of pain. For home use, we think that grounded Velcro body bands, wrapped around the waist, wrist, or knee, will be much more practical.

Pet pads

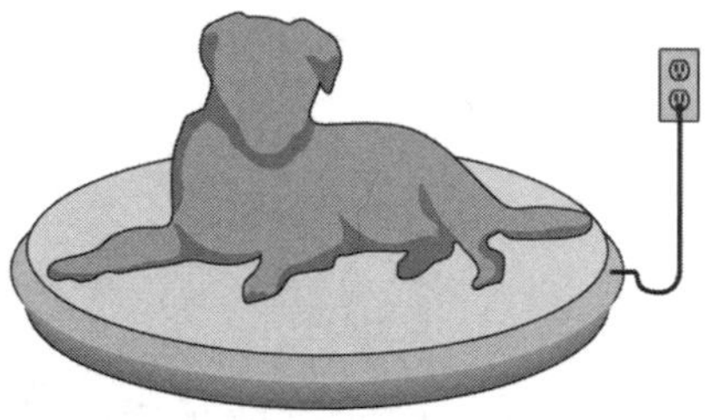

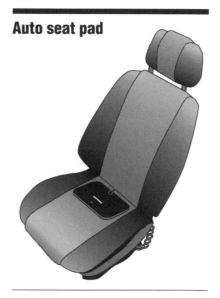

Figure 8-8. Dog on conductive pad.

Earthing Pet Pads

A prototype pad for pets has been tested and found to provide improvement of pain, energy, stamina, flexibility, stress, and old injuries. See Chapter 15 for more details.

Auto seat pad

Auto Seat Pads

A seat pad like this helps ease driver tension and fatigue. Is it a possible remedy for "road rage?" The pad is connected to the metal frame of the vehicle, providing a semi-Earth ground. See Chapter 14 for more details.

Figure 8-9. Conductive auto seat.

CHAPTER 9

A Dozen Years of Earthing: Clint Ober's Observations

Since 1998, I have been invited into the homes of probably several thousand people and reconnected them to the Earth. I have grounded newborns, kids, young adults, midlifers, seniors, and centenarians, and individuals deathly ill for whom the medical system had no more fixes to offer. Some understood what I was doing. Most didn't. They just understood later that they felt better and had less pain.

Earthing produces an amazing grassroots ripple. "Can you please do this for my mother or sister or father or friend?"

I've heard that many times from people who suffered for years with severe pain. Anyone who goes from pain to less pain or no pain, from fatigue to energy, from lack of mobility to more mobility, wants all their loved ones and friends to feel the same way.

"Oh, my God," they will say. "I didn't have to do anything. I didn't have to change my diet or exercise or take a pill. Just go to sleep."

That's what one tells the other, and so the news of Earthing has spread. One woman with MS, who suddenly felt like a new person after grounding herself, told me she wanted to start a "barefoot revolution" and get everybody grounded.

I remember one case in which I grounded a mother at the request of her daughter, whom I had previously grounded. The older woman had suffered from chronic pain in the hips for more than ten years. I placed two grounded electrode patches on her feet. After about twenty minutes or so, she said she had to get up to go to the restroom. So I took the patches off. As she raised herself off the chair, she let out a scream. I got a real scare. I thought something had gone wrong.

"No," she said, "my pain is gone."

Dramatic as that sounds, I've heard it many times over the years. It is simply a common refrain of people being reconnected to the Earth after being disconnected perhaps for a whole lifetime.

The degree of gratification I have had seeing people lose their pain and feel better is beyond description. This is what has kept me going every day on an adventure that has been exhausting, challenging, and at times, quite lonely. My joy has trumped the fatigue and time involved in trying to educate people about Earthing. Again and again, I have witnessed sick and pasty faces turn warm and pink within minutes after someone is connected to the Earth.

After all these years, it is clear beyond any doubt that Earthing is safe and that many conditions and symptoms respond positively to the natural energy of the Earth. It is also clear to me that this connection with the Earth is *the* missing link for restoring red-bloodedness, hardiness, and health back into a society where the level of all of those has been plunging in recent years.

People often ask if Earthing will help them with certain health symptoms.

Just as you can't direct healthy food, air, or water to create specific desired results in one function or part of your body, your body takes the natural energy from the Earth and uses it as needed. Often, people tell me of surprising "side benefits."

I strongly believe also that Earthing is not just to remedy health issues already present, but also to assist our bodies in staying healthy. I have come to think of this as about the most natural form of prevention and anti-aging medicine you can find.

Neither I, nor the researchers and doctors I have worked with over the years, have a full understanding of the depth of physiological changes that occur with Earthing. The research is barely ten years old. I feel we are scratching the surface of a great new paradigm that hopefully others, with greater resources, will be inspired to explore.

This I do know: consistently reconnecting with the Earth restores a natural source of energy to your body that has been missing in your life.

This missing energy may be the core cause of chronic inflammation and pain in your body, a malfunctioning nervous system, or some unresolved personal health issue. When you reconnect, and stay reconnected, all kinds of wonderful things happen.

My observations over the years attest to a seemingly boundless potential for Earthing to help prevent and alleviate both common and uncommon health issues.

COMMON SYMPTOMS THAT IMPROVE

In general, people feel a greater sense of well-being when they are grounded. The sicker the individual, the more striking the gains. Older folks rapidly feel the spark of improved circulation and energy. Color, vitality, and outlook on life are transformed. Swollen joints and varicose veins subside. Some with many health issues are frequently different people after just a week or two of Earthing. Sure, they will still have those same issues, but they are getting better. One or more sources of pain are being reduced. They become more functional. Often they have told me, "I have my life back again."

Many women with menstrual issues have confided to me—a man and a stranger in their lives—that their periods are smoother after they started Earthing. I was once speaking at a health conference and was having a chat with a doctor and his wife afterward. I noticed that the wife had a painful look on her face. I asked her if she was okay. She said openly that it was PMS. I asked her if she would let me see if grounding could help her. I sat her down nearby, where I was demonstrating Earthing, and applied a grounded electrode patch for fifteen minutes on the palm of her hand. At the end of that time, she had a different look on her face. She said most of her discomfort had cleared up. The next day the doctor called me to say that his wife had felt so good that she was exercising on the mini-trampoline in their home. Usually, he said, she was down for a week.

Women in midlife often describe less discomfort from typical hormonal swings with grounding.

The main thing I have seen with children is a rapid calming effect. After grounding kids, parents are usually quite eager to have them traipsing around barefoot in the backyard. Nowadays, the first thing a kid will do in the morning is put on his or her shoes and the last thing at night is take them off. So they are ungrounded pretty much all the time, and this contributes, I believe, to a lot of the new health and emotional problems that kids have today, and it's another factor to add to the list of causes such as junk food, lack of exercise, and being exposed to EMF pollution from long hours of television, computers, and video games.

Many experts are saying that kids—and adults as well—need to get out in Nature more and are healthier and better adjusted if they do so. Stress levels fall within minutes of seeing green spaces, one authority said. I second that, and I would add one more thing: whether you go out into the countryside or your own backyard, go out barefooted wherever safe and possible. The stress level will drop even more.

Earthing helps circulation. That's obvious to me from seeing countless grey faces brighten up with color from better blood flow. The first thing I've noticed—within minutes—with a lot of people is a change in their color. There's more color in their face or extremities. If the extremities are cold, they tend to warm up. "There's something going on down there," people have often told me after ten or fifteen minutes.

People who sleep grounded are calmer, more energetic, and less stressed during the day. They wake up with less stiffness and soreness in the morning.

People with asthma and other respiratory ailments like bronchitis and emphysema breathe better. I've seen this often with children who have asthma.

Headaches often become less intense and frequent, and sometimes go away altogether.

If you have heartburn, go outdoors and plant your feet on the ground for twenty minutes and see what happens. Heartburn and acid reflux benefit from grounding.

Earthing has a stabilizing effect on the nervous system. One striking example of the healing potential on the nervous system was described to me by an acupuncturist who reported that after sleeping Earthed for a year, the mild and infrequent partial seizures she'd had for fifteen years seemed to have stopped.

If you have constipation, grounding may make you regular. It has done so for many people. Some individuals have told me they were able to discontinue having to take laxatives.

I have seen many people with debilitating arthritis who have dramatically improved. I saw this right from the very start.

For individuals who are bedridden, a grounded bed sheet can reduce or eliminate bedsores. Hospitals need to ground their patients!

Eczema and psoriasis improve. So does dry skin. And dry, itchy eyes.

Food and pollen allergies improve and sometimes even clear up. Faulty immune systems seem to work better. By connecting with the Earth, it's as if you press a button on the immune system—like on a computer—that switches disabled to enabled. I know this from firsthand experience. Years ago, when my kids were growing up, they would bring every virus and bug home from school, and I would inevitably catch what they got. In the twelve years since I became grounded, I've had a few colds but that's about it. I used to suffer from pollen allergies, with a particular sensitivity to juniper. When the junipers blossomed, I would have difficulty breathing for weeks. Certain foods would cause red blotches on my throat. If I ate strawberries, I would break out with something like hives. Oranges gave me canker sores. There were long stretches of time when I was living off drugstore allergy remedies just to be somewhat comfortable. One doctor told me to stop eating wheat and grains with gluten. I don't have any of that anymore. I eat everything. I don't have any problem with juniper or pollens.

HOW FAST DOES EARTHING WORK?

There's no guarantee you will have an overnight healing like some of the people in the stories you will soon read about. It may take a while. You won't know until you give it a chance and do it—and stay with it. But I'll tell you this: I have seen plenty of people near death make comebacks that surprised their doctors, or who experienced a better quality of life before they passed away. And people who stay grounded just don't get sick—or as sick as they might normally do. They heal and their energy comes back faster.

People who ground themselves usually say they feel better within an hour, in many cases twenty minutes, whether they are walking or sitting barefooted, or are connected to the Earth through a bed or floor pad, sheet, electrode patch, or grounded shoes. The research shows instant changes in physiology and significant improvements in the body's electrical activity inside a half hour or forty minutes.

I have seen some people with tension headaches have rapid relief, within five minutes. Others, such as someone with a chronic condition like arthritis, may take a half hour or so to notice some level of pain relief. But relief of pain and symptoms, in varying degrees and depending on what condition is involved, is a common response. The speed at which this occurs also varies from person to person. Relief can be significant, overnight, gradual, total, or partial.

I have found that lasting changes in stress, sleep, pain, and body rhythms occur when people are connected to the Earth for longer periods of time on a continual basis. Nighttime sleep, when the body is most receptive to healing, appears to be an ideal time for Earthing. What better time for a healing "treatment" when it occurs effortlessly while you sleep?

WHEN YOU STOP YOU LOSE THE BENEFITS

If you have chronic inflammation and you ground yourself for a period of time, like weeks or months, and then stop, the body will usually sooner or later revert back to its previous ungrounded status. I have seen this regression happen with people and animals alike.

Many people report that the effects of Earthing continue with longer use. It is important not to give up too soon. You are plugging yourself into an energy source that humans have evolved with for millions of years. It is part of Nature's design. Your body's electrical system—that controls every cellular function—will function better when you supply it routinely with what it evolved on.

EARTHING AND MEDICATION

Earthing improves the way the body functions in so many ways and it may, as a result, influence the requirement for medication. A number of people have told me they have been able to reduce their dosage. I advised them, as I do anyone, that if you are involved in any medical treatment program it is best to inform your doctor about grounding. It is highly unlikely that he or she will have any knowledge of Earthing. This is all so relatively new.

If this is your situation you may want to show them this book. In any case, be alert to any symptoms that might reflect a medication overdose. Earthing doesn't interfere with medication. But your doctor may need to adjust the level you are taking. When undergoing routine medical testing, be alert to possible and surprising improvements in your results. Be sure your doctor addresses any changes that occur. Some results may indicate improved functioning and suggest lowering a dosage or even eliminating a medication.

In my experience, grounding can influence thyroid function. Individuals taking thyroid medication should watch for any developing signs of excess dosage. A number of women on thyroid told me they began to experience heart palpitations, a sign of excess thyroid. Once their doctors reduced the dosage, the symptom vanished. The message I gather from these situations is that Earthing may help thyroid function.

Another example is Coumadin, a widely prescribed blood thinner, commonly used in the treatment of patients with cardiovascular conditions. Earthing reduces inflammation, including inflammation in the blood. Inflamed blood is thicker blood, and it's a risk factor for clotting and cardiovascular events. I have seen many people with heart disease benefit from grounding, and our research indicates that Earthing may be extremely beneficial for the heart and blood flow, for instance, by reducing blood thickness and changing in a positive way the bioelectrical dynamics of the blood. I don't really know any contraindications for grounding. After all, what's involved is nothing more than being barefoot on the Earth. However, when it comes to something as critical as Coumadin, we have no direct investigational experience. For this reason, if you are someone taking Coumadin, you should first get your doctor's approval before grounding yourself. If you do decide you would like to ground yourself, it may be prudent to do so for shorter periods in the beginning, such as walking barefoot in the park, or grounding yourself for a few hours in the evening while you watch TV. As you ground yourself, and slowly increase your exposure, monitor your situation and blood more frequently so as to determine if your dosage needs to be lowered. Ground with caution, and have your doctor regularly and carefully check your blood.

EARTHING AND DETOXIFICATION

Some people suffering with chronic inflammation, fibromyalgia, fatigue, anxiety, and depression, or who are taking many pharmaceutical drugs, may feel malaise or flu-like symptoms when they initially ground themselves at night. They may, of course, actually have the flu, which has nothing to do with the effects of Earthing. But if not, it is very likely that the grounding has triggered a detoxification response in the body and promoted the release of toxins. As toxins pass through and out the system, a positive process, you could feel as if you had a flu, with perhaps some nausea or even diarrhea. When this happens, it may be advisable to cut back on the grounding, and start with perhaps an hour a day, and then slowly increase the time.

THE TINGLING SENSATION

People sometimes report feeling a tingling sensation in their body the first few times they are grounded at night. It is not unpleasant. And don't worry: you are not being electrocuted! You are simply feeling the Earth's natural, healing energy coming into your body. The tingling is related to the initial re-energizing, re-synchronizing, and normalizing effects that this transfer of energy generates. The sensation usually diminishes and goes away after a few sessions of Earthing. It may be felt again once the individual resumes Earthing after stopping for some time. Sometimes the energy can create a feeling of achiness in parts of the body that are compromised, for instance, in the legs and feet of patients with diabetes who have poor circulation. As the extremities become energized, the experience initially may be felt as achiness or as fleeting cramps.

THE MALE CONNECTION

A number of men have described having better erections as a result of sleeping grounded. This might be a byproduct of improved circulation. Older men may also experience fewer trips to urinate at night, due likely to reduction of prostate inflammation and deeper sleep.

EARTHING IS DOSE-RELATED

The longer you are able to ground yourself in your daily life, the more stable, energetic, and robust your body functions and the greater your ability to heal. Some people describe symptoms disappearing or improving dramatically after just a few nights of sleeping grounded. Others say that symptoms and energy improve gradually, then reach a plateau and stay at that level as long as they continue grounding themselves. Some, after sleeping grounded through the night, will comment at mid-day that they felt better, had more energy, or less pain when they awoke, but now they don't feel as good.

As far as this last example is concerned, my experience indicates that the person simply needs to be grounded longer—the more time, the better—during the day.

This point was demonstrated dramatically in the case of one young woman who suffered with lupus, an autoimmune disease. She experienced substantial reduction of her symptoms when sleeping grounded for up to eight hours a night. She wanted to feel even better. So she used a grounded floor pad and desk pad at her computer workstation and was able to often log up to eight hours more of Earthing. Her forearms were in contact with the desk pad as she worked, and she took off her shoes while at her desk. The additional hours made a big difference. In her case, Earthing during sleep was good, but sixteen hours of Earthing throughout the whole day was super-good.

The whole thing goes back to Nature and the way our body was designed. We evolved in a grounded state, pretty much 24/7. If you sleep grounded, that's wonderful. That means, though, that your immune system is still in an ungrounded state for sixteen hours a day. I believe that if you can extend your hours of Earthing you stand to benefit even more, particularly if you have serious health issues.

Many individuals have told me about quantum leaps of improvement after extending their grounding hours into their active day. Earthing really has a dose-related effect. The longer you do it, the better.

Dale Teplitz, a health researcher who has worked with me on several of the studies and introduced Earthing to many people, uses a food analogy to help illustrate this point.

"People who eat junk food their entire life are depleted of many essential nutrients," she says. "Their health suffers as a result. If all of a sudden, they eat one healthy meal, they can't expect to have lasting benefits. But if they continue to eat healthy, over time the body gradually takes those elements and creates a healthier person. We humans have been disconnected from the Earth for our whole lives. We are depleted of the health-sustaining energy of the Earth. As with eating healthy, the longer we reconnect with the Earth, the more our body responds with improved health."

A single dose of walking on a sandy beach or sitting barefoot in your backyard will make you feel good for a while, but the effect won't last long. It's another thing if your living situation allows you to pursue those activities on a daily basis. Similarly, if you sleep grounded one night you will sleep better that night and feel more rested in the morning. But if you can routinely sleep grounded you are giving your body a major boost— a rock-solid foundation for maintaining health and a weapon for combating illness. And beyond that, some people will benefit still more from additional hours of grounding, particularly individuals with chronic inflammatory disorders.

Many people have asked over the years if it is harmful to get "too much" of the Earth's energy when grounded. The question is understandable, but there is no evidence of getting too much. To me, it's like asking if a tree is getting too much of the Earth that it is rooted to. We evolved on the Earth and all our ancestors lived with around-the-clock connection with the Earth. It's totally natural to be connected to the Earth and, I think, unnatural and unhealthy not to be connected. Our body knows exactly what to do with what the Earth provides for us. When we connect to the Earth, the amount of the electrons we absorb and utilize is governed by the amount our body needs to balance the bioelectrical state of our body. It is always in the perfect amount. It restores the body's most natural state.

I believe that maximum benefits will come when individuals live grounded around the clock or for a good chunk of a twenty-four-hour period. Our modern world, however, has become largely plasticized and insulated, keeping us separated from the Earth's healing energy. Hopefully, in the near future, we will re-evolve into a grounded society through access to conductive homes, offices, schools, bedding, furniture, and footwear.

Our contemporary fast-paced lifestyle, filled with chronic stress, poor eating choices, and lack of physical activity, has created a sick society. Enjoyment of life is eroded. Personal and governmental resources are hemorrhaged. Earthing doesn't stop the bad habits, but it offers a natural remedy for halting some of the bleeding and the suffering. It is not a do-it-once-and-you-are-cured thing. Nor is it a cure-all. Rather it is a safe, effective, new-old paradigm that truly deserves thorough exploration and exploitation as a primary health and healing tool.

CHAPTER 10

Feedback: What People Say About Earthing

Thousands of people have experienced Earthing. We have invited some of them to share their personal stories in their own words, including doctors and patients, to provide a sampling of the broad and frequently dramatic potential of Earthing.

EARTHING AMBASSADORS

One of the long-time enthusiasts of Earthing is Jim Healy, a leading pioneer in the research, development, and distribution of cutting-edge monitoring, diagnostic, and therapeutic technologies used by doctors and hospitals. Years ago, he participated in designing the first 911 paramedic rescue vehicles and helicopters. He is chairman of Lead-Lok Corp., an international medical products company headquartered in Sandpoint, Idaho. Many people who ground themselves and experience relief for one ailment or another often become "Earthing ambassadors," eager to share Earthing with friends and relatives. Jim is one of them. Here is his story.

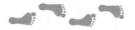

"I've been in the medical instrumentation field for a half-century. In the late 1960s, I started a company specializing in the inspection and upgrading of electrical equipment in hospitals to ensure that the equipment was properly grounded. If not, disturbances or spikes in the electrical current might create a life-threatening shock in a patient connected to a piece of equipment. It was all about grounding the equipment to prevent potential shock. Nobody ever thought that directly grounding a patient could be beneficial.

"When I first heard about Earthing, it made real sense to somebody like me. Clint Ober demonstrated the concept by putting a grounded electrode patch on my leg. The leg was chronically achy. Within twenty minutes, it felt much better. I then started sleeping on grounded sheets. I noticed quickly that I slept better, and all the aches and pains that come with aging improved as well.

"I then began to think of how I could help people close to me. One person I thought of was a friend's daughter who had multiple sclerosis. The results she got from sleeping grounded were unbelievable. She told me she was now able to get up in the morning without her usual aches and pains.

"Some time afterward she came over to see me. She had been on vacation for a month. She said she hadn't taken her grounded sheet with her and was still feeling great, saying, 'as good or better than before when I was sleeping on it.' Now, back at home and sleeping on the grounded sheet again, she wasn't feeling any difference. She wasn't sure the sheet was working anymore.

"I was curious. I asked where she went on vacation. She said Baja California. She and her boyfriend had rented a cottage on the beach. More questioning on my part revealed that for most of the month she never wore shoes. She walked on the sand. She went swimming and snorkeling.

"'That's the whole point,' I told her. 'You *were* grounding yourself every day. Walking barefoot on the Earth. Swimming in saltwater. That's super grounding.'

"'Is that the same thing,' she asked?

"'Absolutely,' I told her. 'There is nothing magical about the grounded sheet or the bed pad connected to a wall plug or ground rod. It is all about getting back to Nature and reconnecting to the Earth one way or another. You get the same effect barefoot on the beach or in the park or your backyard garden or sleeping on a grounded bed pad. The more hours you do it, the better.'

"She then wanted to know if Earthing might help her mother who had painful rheumatoid arthritis, particularly in the knees. Her mother, she said, put two Advils on her nightstand every evening. When she woke up in the morning, she would take the pills, wait an hour or so until they went to work in her body, and then finally get out of bed. Otherwise her legs hurt too much.

"I heard back that after a couple of days of sleeping grounded, her mother wasn't taking the pills anymore. She was getting up in the morning without pain, and needless to say was very happy about it. Now, her husband, who was my friend, is a medical professional and a real skeptic. He was observing all this and seeing how it had helped his wife and daughter. He was very surprised about their improvement and then reluctantly told me his own story. He had had a bad left shoulder for years and because of the pain only slept on his right side. After sleeping for a while on the grounded sheet that his wife had put on the bed, he noticed that he was now sleeping on his left side without any pain.

"Then there's the story of an acupuncturist in town. One day, she and I were talking. She said she hadn't been riding her bicycle lately because of pain in one foot. She had treated herself but hadn't gotten any relief. So I gave her some electrode patches with a ground connection and said to give it a try. The following day she called all excited. She couldn't believe it. Her pain was gone. So she then invited some of her patients to sit grounded for a half hour with an electrode patch attached to wherever they had pain. She wasn't charging them for it. The women were coming in three times a week, sitting there, and getting pain relief. I told the acupuncturist that if they would just walk barefoot in their gardens for the same amount of time they would get the same results as they would in her office. There is nothing magical about the current in the wire coming out of the wall. Most people just don't understand the simplicity of grounding.

"I also gave a bed pad to one of my company directors, a man who suffers with multiple sclerosis. He was also a skeptic. I asked him about it a couple of weeks later and he shrugged it off, saying he gave the pad to his daughter who has some aches and pains. He said he felt he was too far gone to get any help. A week later, he said his daughter had given it back to him and he decided to try it anyway. He had slept with it for three or four nights, and he said he couldn't believe the results and that much of his pain was gone. He was walking better. His legs didn't collapse as often. He still has MS, but his symptoms are greatly reduced. He walks without as much pain and is much more comfortable."

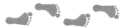

"I Wouldn't Go Anywhere without My Sheets": Another Earthing ambassador is Donna Tisdale, a top Nashville real estate broker.

"Where do I start?" she said when asked about her Earthing experience.

"Let me start with allergies. I have been plagued with miserable seasonal allergies all my life. As a real estate professional, I'd be out showing property, and I would sneeze maybe ten or fifteen times in a row. I would laugh and tell my clients I'm allergic to the months of May and September. Well, it's been a year since I started sleeping grounded. First May came and went, and then September, and guess what? I have not taken one allergy med the entire spring and summer! I've sneezed maybe a few times and that's it. I have not gotten up one single solitary time in the middle of the night to clear my sinuses so I could breathe and sleep! This has been unbelievable.

"For fifteen years, I've had a weird autoimmune skin disease called granuloma annulare. It produces unsightly breakouts on my legs, arms, and trunk. Now it's almost completely gone on my arms, and almost completely gone on my legs. It's amazing. I've been to dermatologists all over the place, and nobody has a cure for it or knows what causes it.

"My eighty-eight-year-old mother has been incontinent for fifteen years. She had bladder surgery, and it didn't work. So she would use fifteen to twenty pads a day. She came to visit for a month six weeks after she started to sleep grounded. She was now using maybe one or two pads a day. 'I think it's the sheets,' she said.

"She also had shoulder pain for three years from an injury and could not raise her right hand over her shoulder. One day during her visit I saw her combing her hair with her right hand. I asked her about it. She said, 'My shoulder doesn't hurt anymore. I think it's the sheets.'

"For three years, my husband Bill was looking at knee surgery and getting injections into the knees. He's passed on the shots now because the knees aren't hurting as bad. At a family wedding over Labor Day weekend in 2009, we danced together for the first time in years. His knees are doing great. He has also suffered with plantar fasciitis, and now that is totally gone. One of my sisters had that as well. It would come and go.

She's been sleeping grounded and now hasn't had a single flare-up in months.

"Another sister has very aggressive rheumatoid arthritis. She's sleeping grounded and says she has very few flare-ups anymore.

"A dear friend who has Lyme disease used to have as many as fifteen migraine headaches a month and now she has one or two. She went to Arizona to visit her mom for a week. She forgot to take the sheets with her. She had four migraines during that time. I told her she was crazy. I wouldn't go anywhere without my sheets.

"From the start, we slept much better on the grounded sheets. Bill stopped getting up three times at night like he used to do. He and his bladder are seventy years old. A few weeks after we started sleeping grounded, we headed off on a weekend trip out-of-state to visit family. I wanted to take the sheets. Bill didn't. I gave in. Well, he flipped and he flopped at night. He was up. He was down. He didn't sleep well. So when we went to Austin to see the grandchildren for Christmas, guess what? We took the sheets! We slept well. Now we don't go anywhere without them.

"Do I ever have a passion for getting people Earthed!"

THE SPIRITUAL CONNECTION

Gabriel Cousens, M.D., sixty-seven, Patagonia, Arizona, director of Tree of Life Rejuvenation Center: "I applied Earthing first to myself and my wife. We both felt a difference. Our sleep is deeper. We used to go barefoot some of the time. Now we go barefoot all the time.

"In my work, I am on the go all day long. Now I find myself getting up earlier than before, and despite a half hour or an hour less sleep than I normally used to get, I have more energy. I've always been a high-energy person, but now I have more.

"My clinical impression is that Earthing helps decrease inflammation in people with autoimmune disorders. I have seen it make a difference for people with depression and anxiety. At the Tree of Life Rejuvenation Center, we recommend that everyone who comes here for treatment sleeps on grounding sheets, and everyone benefits in some way or another. People are more relaxed, sleep better, and have more energy as a result.

"Beyond these things, Earthing represents a whole way of thinking. It really speaks to the problem today that people on this planet have lost touch with the Earth and have not returned to the Earth. They have gotten further and further away. From a biblical perspective, people who lose touch with the Earth lose touch with God. There is a whole deeper understanding here. Earthing reconnects us to the Earth, to others, and, in a sense, to God."

THE MOST BENEFITS FOR LEAST AMOUNT OF WORK

David Wolfe, thirty-nine, San Diego, speaker and author on healthy lifestyle: "Personally, I've seen three surprising changes after I started Earthing two years ago. The first was the disappearance of a stubborn remnant of an infection—likely one of those antibiotic-resistant staph infections. I developed the infection on my big toe about eight years ago and battled it for a couple of years, down to one lump that looked like scar tissue. Occasionally, it would bother me. I used all the healing tools at my disposal and even asked for help from some health professionals I know. But I couldn't eliminate it. Then I started using a grounded floor pad as I worked on my computer or on the telephone. Within two days, the lump was gone. Like magic.

"Similarly, I had a very sensitive tooth for about twenty-five years. I had cracked it at age fourteen. The tooth was sensitive to cold water and any kind of sugar or sweetener. If I chewed down on a small, hard object like a seed and it pressed against the tooth, there would be a jolt of pain. After a few months of Earthing, I noticed the sensitivity disappeared.

"The biggest change health-wise has been with my allergies. As a kid, they were completely disruptive. I was extremely sensitive to cats and pollen, especially ragweed. Exposure could incapacitate me for two or three days. In pollen season, my lungs would fill with mucus and fluid. I would get intense itchiness in my eyes, ears, and back of the throat. My eyes would tear. The allergies have gotten better over the years as I have improved my nutrition. But Earthing has been like the coup de grace. I've gone through two pollen allergy seasons now without any problem. No symptoms. If I go into a house now where a cat resides, I am good for about an hour. Before I couldn't even go into the house.

"Besides the changes in me, I have seen and heard pretty amazing things when other people are grounded. One woman who came to one of my health seminars was in obvious pain. She was sitting in the front row, and I could see her discomfort written on her face. I went over and asked her about it. She said she suffered with back pain for twenty years. I had a grounding pad with me. I connected it into a wall outlet and she put it inside her blouse against her back. An hour and twenty minutes later, when I finished my talk, her face had totally changed. She couldn't believe what had happened. She said her pain was gone. I was shocked. Everybody in the room was shocked.

"Pretty much everybody who sleeps grounded says they sleep better. One interesting feedback I've gotten from a number of people is that they feel different when they work grounded at their computers. They describe the feeling with words like 'comfort,' 'security,' and 'safety.' A few of them have said they actually don't like working at a computer anymore unless they are grounded.

"In my work as a health educator and speaker, I focus on what's natural, good for healing, and good for people in general. I'm also very much attuned to what is the least amount of work that somebody can do and get the most benefits. That's a number one consideration for me because in the health world people want to get the most benefits for the least amount of work. Well, it became clear to me after about a month of Earthing that this was it. Earthing gives you the most benefits for the least amount of work of anything I've ever seen. There is no work!"

IMPROVING THE LIFE OF A DOCTOR AND HIS PATIENTS

David Gersten, M.D., sixty, Encinitas, California, practitioner of nutritional medicine and integrative psychiatry: "A few years ago, I developed what I called a 'cause and effect' health map that plots out why people get sick with chronic illness and stay sick. I narrowed it down to a simple three-step process. In all chronic illness, you have primary causes (level one), which includes genetics, infections, toxins, digestive problems and malabsorption, and mental, emotional, and stress factors. Level two involves how the body reacts to these primary causes, namely through inflammation and the stress response. Level three relates to total body disturbances of biochemistry, or what I call metabolic chaos. Over time, it has become clear to me that Earthing has a profound healing effect on level two.

"I've been grounded for about three years, and now it's completely integrated into my practice. I see people all the time who come to a doctor like me as a last resort. The first feedback I usually hear after a patient starts Earthing is an email the following morning that says, 'I just had the best sleep in twenty years.'

"I provided a grounding unit to a ninety-six-year-old friend who had severe osteoarthritis for probably twenty-five years. I didn't explain a word to her. I just explained it to her son. After a few days, I called to see how she was doing. He said his mother, a well-known folk medicine healer in San Diego for decades, told him her pain was down more than three-quarters. But what was really amazing was that her passion for life had come back. She had had a stroke six months before, and although she had recovered from the physical effects, she had lost her typical passion for life. This was a vital woman who was still traveling and giving lectures. 'It's back,' her son told me.

"People frequently come to me for chronic fatigue syndrome (CFS), a problem that often involves cognitive issues like memory, concentration, focus, and brain fog. One such patient was a sixty-five-year-old woman. She had had CFS, plus hypertension, for a very long time. I told her to get grounded. On day thirty-one after she started, she emailed me to say her energy was much improved from the Earthing but also her cognition had suddenly returned. Moreover, her blood pressure numbers had dropped and began to quickly normalize. I advised her to monitor her blood pressure carefully each day. She had been taking two blood pressure medications that another doctor had prescribed. Her blood pressure came down so fast that on her own, without consulting with me, she discontinued one of the blood pressure meds. She then went back to her other doctor, who prescribed a much weaker prescription. Now, along with the Earthing, she is able to maintain a normal blood pressure. Her fatigue and most of her other CFS symptoms have vastly improved.

"In terms of my own personal experiences, I didn't see anything miraculous, at least not for a while. For decades, I have suffered with keratoconus, a condition in which the cornea of the eye becomes progressively thin, leading to significant visual loss. About one out of two thousand people in the population have this problem. The cornea thins out and blows out like a balloon, and you can't get a contact to fit on it anymore. I've had five corneal transplants over the years. Three in the right eye were rejected, resulting in considerable inflammation and the formation of hundreds of minute blisters on the surface of the cornea. In the latter stages of rejection, the pain is absolutely agonizing. I was a good year and a half into the rejection of my 2004 transplant when I began to ground myself. In addition to the pain, I was waking up each morning with drainage coming out of the eye. After about four months of Earthing, I woke up one morning and realized that the drainage was not there. From that day on, there has been no drainage at all. The pain level has stayed low, and it's very tolerable almost all the time. I do still have occasional to rare days when the pain is high enough to require a strong painkiller. But now I'm three years into a rejection that would not have been bearable without Earthing. This is a good thing for me because I need to wait for stem cell research before I have another corneal transplant.

"In any case, I have no vision out of the right eye. Although I haven't had the corneal transplant rejection issue with the left eye, I was definitely losing vision in that eye and was quite concerned to say the least. I had been going downhill for about fifteen years until I started Earthing. Then the vision loss stopped and reversed. My optometrist was amazed at the dramatic improvement in vision. I asked him if he had ever seen anyone who had a degenerative eye disease that suddenly reversed after decades. He said he had never seen that before. For me, this was pretty miraculous.

"Another personal experience made me keenly aware of the power of Earthing. I was working at night in a clinic and had stepped outside to take a short break. While outside, I walked smack into a metal post with a 'No Parking' sign. The side of the post was like a dull knife blade, and it put a half-inch gash in my forehead down to the bone. It was bleeding badly. I ran back into the clinic and had my nurse clean the wound and bandage it up. I would have sent any patient with this kind of cut to the emergency room. But I had more patients to see. The next day, I pulled off the bandages and there was just a small line, like a small surgical incision, where the cut was. There was no sign of redness, heat, swelling, or pain. There was virtually no inflammation. On day two, I could just make out the edges of the gash. The edges of the cut were starting to come together and heal. On day six, it was so completely healed that there was no sign of the cut at all.

"I was also impressed by the experience of a patient who, in addition to CFS, suffered with anxiety. Immediately after she grounded herself, she had a significant decrease in her anxiety. Her overall health and energy improved. What made the most impact on me was what she described as a sense of renewed connectedness to the Earth, to others around her, and to the absolute core of her being. She felt this connectedness so much when she was grounded that she took her bed pad with her to work. She slept on it at night and used it at her desk during the day. She said she was experiencing her deepest self, 'a new me,' she called it, without all the worry, the fear, the anxiety, and the restless mind. 'I'm changed at the core,' she said.

"The feedback I have from patients is now so strong that I know pre-dictably, as a doctor, this will change a person's life. Maybe three out of nearly one hundred patients have said they didn't notice any difference."

THE ANTI-AGING CONNECTION

With the passage of time, changes inexorably occur in the human body. The signs of aging range from the obvious—weight gain, loss of height, muscular weakness—to the hidden—loss of elasticity in blood vessels, slowdown in hormonal output, and most significantly, cellular damage from unrelenting free-radical activity. Doctors see a wide variety of phys-iological responses to the aging process. Some eighty-year-old individuals physically appear to be fifty or sixty. Conversely, some middle-aged peo-ple in their forties and fifties look like they are ready for retirement. There are many reasons why some people "age" faster than others. Could Earth-ing be one ingredient for slowing down the process?

Growing older is inevitable. Anti-aging strategies are not about living to one hundred or one hundred and twenty, but about growing older grace-fully and with energy. The goal is to prevent illness and develop physical and mental potential in the pursuit of satisfaction and aliveness.

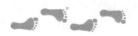

Arvord Belden, Ph.D., ninety, Yountville, California, retired clinical psychologist: "I've been sleeping grounded pretty regularly for more than eight years. Within a year, I realized that I wasn't going to doctors like I used to do. My hands and hip hurt me less from arthritis. I also noticed that my mind seems to be clearer, and I seem to have more energy and stamina.

"After a year, I had a checkup with my doctor, and he commented that he was amazed at my excellent health given my age.

"Now after all these years of continued Earthing, I can't say I've reversed the aging process. I still have the arthritis, but I don't need to take any medication for it. In fact, I don't take a single medication for anything. I feel darn good for somebody who is ninety. My energy is great.

"I still do a lot of yard work, including tree pruning, and I've had my share of cuts, scrapes, and even falls. I was out a few weeks ago on my recumbent three-wheeler bike and I took a fall. I banged myself up but didn't break anything, and I healed up nice and quick. Same thing with the yard work. None of the cuts ever get infected, even though I don't put any topical medicine on them.

"My sleep has definitely been better ever since I started this. If I wake up at night, it seems like after a minute or so, I am back sleeping again."

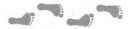

Katherine Van Hatten, seventy-one, Brentwood, California, massage therapist, acupressurist: "I've been working and sleeping grounded for five years. I still work a full day, and the only way I can do that at my age, without going home exhausted, is to stand barefoot on a floor pad that is grounded while I give my massages. If I don't use it, I can do maybe one or two massages a day. If I work on the pad, I can work a full day, meaning four, five, or even six massages. Moreover, my clients receive the benefit because for the whole hour that they're on the table I am bringing free electrons to them through the pad, my body, and my hands. So they are grounded as well.

"A new client once told me she never had such a good night's sleep in her life as she did after the massage. Ever since I have been working grounded my clients tell me routinely that they experience a higher level of energy afterward for an extended period of time.

"I'm also an acupressure therapist, so between that and massage, my hands and wrists are working hard with a lot of pressure. Until I grounded myself, I quite often experienced fatigue and muscle pain. I feel that the regeneration from sleeping grounded and also working while standing on a grounded floor pad is really giving me extra years to work.

"In my profession, there's a tremendous amount of burn out because the work is very physical. You use a lot of energy. I've been at this for twenty-four years, and even if I go home tired now, I go to bed, sleep on the bed pad and get up and I'm ready to go. And my husband has experienced the same thing. He stopped snoring the first night he was on the pad. We have been able to sleep fabulously."

ARTHRITIS

The most prevalent form of arthritis is osteoarthritis, also known as degenerative joint disease, wear-and-tear arthritis, or just plain arthritis. The incidence increases with age. Rheumatoid arthritis (RA) differs from osteo in that it is an autoimmune disease, the result of the immune system attacking the body's own tissue. RA can affect other body parts besides joints, such as the eyes, mouth, and lungs. Of these two common forms of arthritis, RA is the most inflammatory. Either one causes pain, stiffness, and can lead to inactivity and disability.

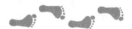

Sheila Curtiss, sixty-three, San Diego, sales: "I was born unhealthy. I'm amazed that I'm alive now. If it weren't for Earthing, I'm not sure I would be.

"I used to have scary episodes of heart fibrillation. They stopped shortly after I started grounding myself and haven't returned. The constant hot flashes I had been experiencing for some years stopped within the first month of grounding.

"But it was the effect on my rheumatoid arthritis that made the biggest and quickest impression on me. I had bad pain and swelling in both knees, particularly the left, and was kind of hobbling all the time. I would have flare-ups from time to time, and with each episode, it seemed like they were getting worse. The one knee was so swollen I could barely get my leg into my pants. I'd have to lift my leg to get into the car. And all my other joints popped and cracked. Elbows. Wrists. Shoulders. When you hear your joints pop, you wonder what's going on? Am I going to break something?

"I knew one of the top orthopedic surgeons in the area and consulted with him. He told me I should have knee surgery in the next six to eight weeks and until then be careful because my knee could lock up on me. I might fall and hurt myself. He wanted to do more testing, but I never had it done. I was reluctant to have a lot of testing because of negative experiences in the past.

"The following weekend I heard Clint Ober speak at a health conference. His idea sounded interesting to me and I decided to follow up immediately. I got grounded. And in three weeks, the pain and swelling were gone. Where did they go? All I know is that they were gone. Gradually, over time all my joints quit popping.

"I've been grounded since 2000, and it has made such a big impact on my health that I stay grounded all the time. People began calling me the barefoot lady. Right now, as I am speaking to you on the phone, I'm standing outside barefoot on my lawn. And when I'm by my computer I have a grounded footpad. When I sit to watch TV, I also have a footpad. And I sleep grounded. The only time I'm not grounded is walking from point A to point B, but maybe that will change when they start making grounded shoes.

"Now, years later, I'm doing really well for somebody my age. I hike, walk, and exercise, probably not as much as I should, but I'm able to do it without any problem. I can move freely. I have become addicted to Earthing. I love the feeling and can tell the difference when I am not grounded."

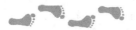

Howell Runion, Ph.D., seventy-six, Stockton, California, former professor of neurophysiology: "I have rheumatoid arthritis involving my hands, shoulders, lumbar area, and lower extremities. There is nothing going to remove this disorder. It is progressive and degenerative. I've had the condition for eight or so years and it has been slowly progressing. I take a lot of medication to manage this and some other problems.

"A friend for whom I have a lot of respect told me about Earthing at night, and I tried it and noticed there was a tremendous difference. I thought at first it was just my imagination. I stopped using it. The condition got worse again. So I tried it again, and I felt better. Nevertheless, I still thought it might be my imagination. But it wasn't my imagination. It did make a difference—a significant decrease in discomfort. It became clear to me that when I don't sleep grounded, I don't feel as good as when I do. I get up the next morning much more refreshed. If I don't use it for several days, I can tell the difference. I feel worse.

"On a scale of 1 to 10, where 10 is so bad that you wish you had something to blow your brains out, my pain level without sleeping grounded is often around 8. Sleeping grounded, the level may be about 5. This is not a cure. But it certainly helps, and the difference makes it worth doing. I believe there is a slowing of deterioration.

"For anyone who suffers from rheumatoid arthritis, I recommend this simple, effective procedure of sleeping on a grounded sheet as an aid to significant pain reduction. It works!"

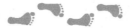

Steve Garner, fifty-two, West Valley City, Utah, auto technician: "Working on cars for a living is brutal on the hands and body. But that's what I was doing for years until rheumatoid arthritis put me out of action.

"In 1993, I was diagnosed with RA after developing a lot of pain in my hands, ankles, and knees. For the next twelve years, I went to the rheumatology clinic at a university medical center every three months for treatment and evaluation. They put me on six different prescription drugs during that time. Each one had side effects that I couldn't live with.

"One medication I received was called diclofenac. The side effects were terrible: headaches, dizziness and my guts feeling like they wanted out. I told the doctor that this was not the drug for me. She then prescribed methotrexate but warned me that it could also cause a lot of side effects. It sure did. After about a week, the pain had gone down quite a bit and the inflammation was a little better, but I felt like I had a constant cold with a runny nose, head congestion, and headaches. These were just some of the side effects.

"Meanwhile, my sleep was disturbed from the pain and my performance at work was suffering. The disease was taking the fun and purpose out of my life. I began taking massive amounts of ibuprofen. I started with 200 to 500 milligrams (mg). This was just barely taking down the pain and very little of the inflammation. I increased the daily doses to as much as 3,000 mg. I lived like this for five years.

"In 2005, I was forced to retire because of the constant pain and inflammation in my hands. It was impossible to continue my work.

"A couple of years before, I had been given a grounded bed pad as a gift, but I was too skeptical. I stashed it in the closet. It sounded too weird to me. After the pain forced me to stop working, I was willing to try anything. I found the bed pad in the closet and started sleeping grounded.

"I only wish I had done that before. I experienced a change after the very first night. I had the best night's sleep in years! The inflammation and pain eased a lot within a few days, and after four weeks the pain was gone!

"Awhile later, I went back to see my doctor. She was impressed with the improvement in my overall heath. She told me that the improvement showed in my face. She said that I looked like a new person. She did x-rays on my hands and could not find any inflammation. She commented that the new medications must have been really working. When I told her that I had not been taking any of the medications but just sleeping grounded, she looked puzzled. I told her I was going to keep doing it. And I have.

"Today, four years later, I am still pain free and I have not had to take even so much as an aspirin. This thing has literally changed my life! I have felt so good that I was able to return to work. I am now back turning wrenches again."

AUTISM

Autism is a complex developmental disability that affects an individual's ability, in different ways and degrees, to communicate and interact with others. It typically shows up during the first three years of life and is not outgrown, causing a potentially severe emotional and financial burden on families for decades. There is no known single cause for this condition, which has risen steeply in recent years. The Centers for Disease Control and Prevention (CDC) estimates it affects one out of every 150 American children. The Autism Society of America says the lifetime cost of caring for an individual with autism ranges from $3.5 to $5 million. Typical signs of autism include lack of or delay of spoken language, repetitive use of language and/or motor mannerisms (e.g., hand-flapping, twirling objects, little or no eye contact, lack of interest in peer relationships, lack of spontaneous or make-believe play, and persistent fixation on parts of objects). Sleep disturbance is often a major problem and can profoundly disrupt normal family routines.

Earthing is not a cure for autism, but over the years it's been seen to have a calming effect, improve sleep patterns, and promote better speech and socializing. Reducing the impact of autism on a child in this natural and simple way simultaneously lessens the stress level in the whole family. Earthing opens a door of hope.

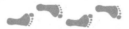

Ron Petruccioni, forty-four, Anaheim, California, businessman: "My daughter Rosanna, fourteen, was diagnosed with moderate autism. Her condition presents itself mostly as an expressive and receptive language disorder. She often cannot produce the words fast enough and stumbles or mumbles her speech. I sometimes have to tell her, 'What did you say? Slow down!' Or in new situations and social environments where she is having some anxiety, she might mix up her tenses and switch inappropriately from first to third person when speaking about herself or others.

"Rosanna has slept on a grounded bed pad since early 2008. We also placed a grounded desk pad at her computer, where she spends an hour or two each day. So she has been getting in some extra daily grounding time.

"Within about a month after being grounded, I started to see her calmer. Her speech became more understandable. That alone has been a great improvement and stress reliever for both of us. There was less frustration showing. The anxiety wasn't there. Occasionally, I will have to tell her to slow down, but not nearly as much as before.

"She has also been sleeping better. She's been easier to wake up.

"Over the years in school, there has been an aide or teacher's assistant assigned to monitor her. Within a short period of time after Rosanna was grounded, the aide noted in her logbook that my daughter participates more actively in the class. Lunch with the kids was more enjoyable for her, and the other kids were engaging her more.

"This makes me so happy. These are subtle things that can't be determined by a lab test. Rosanna is now in the eighth grade, in a mainstream class, and for the first time, there is nobody assigned to keep an eye on her. This is a big deal. She seems happier, more confident, with a little higher self-esteem. She has continued to slowly, smoothly, and surely improve.

"Everyone involved in this disorder knows that autism is a marathon, not a sprint. But what happened in a couple of months and has continued is a miracle for me. A cloud has lifted a bit, and I can think ahead to high school. Maybe college? And to see her become a productive member of society? That's a possibility. High school is a given now. There's hope. And that's huge.

"What I really like about this is that it is so very easy to use. With the autistic community, it's often very hard to find something effective. This is not about how many supplements you can get down them or rubbing on some cream. You just put a grounded pad on a bed, and there are real therapeutic benefits for hardly any cost. A lot of us parents are really strapped, emotionally, physically, and financially. This is something special."

Autism: Meltdowns and Moodiness Much Improved

One California mother said her five-year-old son was diagnosed with autism two years before. She described her situation thusly: "He used to wake up bright-eyed around 5:30 a.m. Then he would 'burnout' from not enough sleep in the late afternoon or early evening. It was like hitting the wall. Crying. Meltdowns. Moodiness.

"We have had him sleeping on the grounded bed pad for seven months, and he now sleeps much more soundly and for a full eleven hours without waking up. I now realize that my son was just sleep deprived, which

Ron Petruccioni's Earthing Survey

In 2009, Ron Petruccioni, the father of a teenage daughter with autism, contacted parents with autistic children around the country for the purpose of participating in an informal study involving Earthing. The idea was to provide interested parents with a grounded bed pad and have their children sleep grounded for a two-month period. The parents were asked to initially complete a twenty-question survey before the experiment and then answer the same questions on a weekly basis until the experiment ended. The questions for the survey were prepared by Mr. Petruccioni, in conjunction with a Southern California mental health expert. A total of twenty-eight parents, whose children ranged in age from two to thirteen, participated in the project. The average age of the youngsters was six for girls and seven for boys. The results included the following (in percentages):

	% Before	% After
Will say goodbye		
Almost always	17.9	27.9
Almost never	46.4	23.4
Responds to familiar people		
Almost always	17.9	24.4
Almost never	32.1	15.7
Is drawn to other children		
Most of the time	17.9	33.0
Almost never	53.6	22.8
When upset, screams rather than cries tears		
Almost always	35.7	21.8
Almost never	7.1	4.1
Watches other children when they are around		
Almost always	10.7	10.2
Almost never	42.9	18.3
Actions are impulsive		
Almost always	35.7	17.8
Almost never	10.7	21.3

	% Before	% After
Has multiple allergies		
Almost always	50.0	21.8
Almost never	21.4	21.3
Likes being touched by caregivers		
Almost always	17.9	13.2
Most times	21.4	33.0
Almost never	39.3	16.2
Uses grunts or crying to communicate needs		
Almost always	17.9	18.8
Sometimes	21.4	39.1
Almost never	39.3	17.3
Sleep is calm and not restless		
Almost always	3.6	14.2
Almost never	53.6	21.8
Easygoing and flexible in schedule		
Almost always	3.6	11.7
Almost never	39.3	18.3
Easily angered		
Almost always	32.1	17.3
Almost never	7.1	16.8

we all know is an issue in itself. The pad is wonderful. He is much improved, primarily due to the pad along with dietary and environmental changes we have made.

"Hardly anybody would know there are or have been autistic type issues with him. The only problems are a speech delay (about one and one-half to two years behind his peers) and some residual allergies.

"In addition to sleeping grounded, our son always goes barefooted. He loves it. You should see that kid run over our landscape rocks. He has feet of steel."

BACK PAIN

Mary Mason, sixty-six, Colfax, California, retired oncology nurse: "I suffered with bad back pain for twenty-five years. It was something I had to live with because you can't take narcotic painkillers and work with patients. You have to be very clear-headed. So Tylenol was my drug of choice. That was it.

"As a nurse, I was skeptical about this Earthing idea when I first heard about it. But I decided to give it a try, and I'm sure glad I did. I've been sleeping grounded for four years and wouldn't think of sleeping any other way. Within two or three days, I noticed a difference. I remember calling my daughter at the end of the first week and telling her that my back wasn't hurting anymore.

"I don't have back pain as long as I sleep on the bed pad. It was proven to me very graphically once when I went to visit my daughter in Florida for two weeks. I didn't take the pad, and that trip home on the plane was excruciating. As soon as I got back home, I got myself onto the pad and the pain eased away.

"Another time I washed the pad and forgot to put it on the bed that night. When you're pain free, you don't think about it. I left it drying on the chair on the patio and woke up the next morning with pain. So I took a nap on the pad and got rid of the pain.

"Now I use it religiously and take it with me no matter where I go. Nothing has ever worked for me like that. It has really helped my quality of life overall.

"From my perspective as someone who worked with ill patients for more than twenty-five years, I think that Earthing could help so many patients. You could eliminate many problems and speed the healing process. Today, they give you one pill for one thing and then another one for the side effects. And it goes on ad nauseam. Earthing could eliminate a lot of that. It could be extremely helpful in surgical recovery and chronic pain clinics."

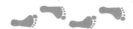

Anita Pointer, sixty-one, Beverly Hills, California, singer: "Throughout my adult life, I have had on-and-off lower back pain. I always travel a lot in connection with my work as a singer. But long flights and pull - ing suitcases around often bring out the pain. Sleeping grounded has helped a lot with the problem. After a recent trip, for instance, I returned home in pain. I was also feeling fatigued and a bit low. I slept on the sheets that night, and the next day the pain was gone, plus I had a lot of fresh energy and my mood was much lighter. Sleeping grounded has also helped improve elimination. I feel this is really doing some good for me."

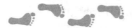

Jim Bellacera, fifty-one, Rocklin, California, business motivational speaker: "Six years ago, I first heard about sleeping on a bed pad that was grounded. I thought I would be a great test case because for more than twenty plus years I had had chronic pain from my days in construction and cabinetmaking. My pain problems started at around age twenty-six. I had back pain, neck pain, and carpal tunnel pain. During one job, I jumped off a trailer while carrying one of my cabinets, and I crushed my back. And that act alone caused me to have endless and serious pain.

"Nothing I ever did ever seemed to help, from seeing doctors and get- ting regular back treatments to taking 800 mg of ibuprofen two or three times a day and sometimes other anti-inflammatories as well.

"And, son of a gun, I woke up in disbelief the morning after the first night I slept grounded. 'No, this can't be,' I said. 'My back doesn't hurt.'

"Not only didn't it hurt, but after a day or two, I didn't have to reach for my daily dose of big ibuprofen horse pills.

"Getting up in the mornings was also a challenge. Before I would roll out of bed, use my arms, and do kind of a push-up with my feet touch- ing the ground so I could stand straight up without bending my back. That changed right away with the grounded pad. You can't believe what it meant to be able to get out of bed with no pain. Today, I don't have pain in the back, neck, or wrists. It's been an absolute blessing.

"Anybody who's in business for themselves is feeling a lot of different types of stresses. There are a lot of things going in your mind 24/7. You're never really turned off. So for me, one of the hardest things to do was just actually going to sleep. It used to be where I would just toss and turn all the time, and my head would go back and forth, until at some point I would fall asleep. Besides the pain, I also noticed from the start that I went to sleep really fast and I'd wake up in the morning really refreshed and with more energy."

INFLAMMATION OF THE BLOOD VESSELS

Behcet's syndrome causes problems in many parts of the body, including skin sores, swelling of parts of the eyes, pain, swelling and stiffness of joints, meningitis, blood clots, inflammation of the digestive system, and blindness. The condition mostly affects people in their twenties and thirties. There is no cure. Treatment focuses on reducing pain and preventing serious problems.

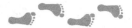

Randy Gillett, fifty-five, Upland, California, retired manager of bedding manufacturing company: "In December of 1999, I was diagnosed with Behcet's syndrome. Within seventy-two hours of becoming ill, I was left profoundly deaf and in a constant state of vertigo, a result of lack of blood flow to my inner ears and vestibular (balance) centers caused by inflammation.

"I also lost sight in one eye and had constant joint pain throughout my body, especially in my blistered and swollen feet. I developed ulcers in my mouth and lesions on various parts of my body, and I was left extremely fatigued.

"After months of medications and bed rest, I was able to return to work, but I still had to take multiple medications to reduce inflammation and regulate my immune system.

"At the end of each work week, I would be very fatigued and spent most of my weekends sleeping. My feet got progressively worse with pain and swelling. I had to start wearing sandals to work and kept a pair of house slippers by my desk to wear around the office. My doctor prescribed Vioxx for the pain and inflammation in my feet. I fully expected that some day I would not be able to walk, and chronic pain was something I must live with. Between the medications and pain, I would be up three to six times a night and sometimes couldn't sleep at all.

"I started sleeping on a grounded pad in February 2004. In the morning, after the third night of sleeping grounded, my feet were no longer swollen. I was able to wiggle my toes and didn't have any pain. It was unbelievable. Every morning after that was like waking up with new feet. I was able to stop taking the prednisone, the Vioxx, and a blood-thinning medication. I was sleeping deeper than ever before and most of the time completely through the night. On weekends, instead of sleeping, I was able to enjoy my leisure time.

"Ear cochlear implant surgery, along with behind-the-ear sound enhancement technology, has helped my hearing on one side, although it is nowhere near what God gave me. I do not expect the grounding to restore my hearing and cure the vertigo or completely restore the damage done to my body by Behcet's, but I know it has reduced the pain caused by inflammation, and in fact, I wake up pain free every morning.

"I sleep grounded every night and will always do so. It keeps the inflammation in check and helps me to be as healthy as possible. Because of grounding I am able to function pretty good and have had very few flare-ups.

"I still see my doctor every four months and get blood work done every year. My doctor tells me my blood tests are like that of a man in his thirties. Now, that is really something since I am fifty-five.

"I tried working for five years after getting better, but I was withdrawing from people, accounts, and phone calls. Doing everyday business was just too stressful. The amount of energy and focus to try and stay balanced and understand what was being said was exhausting, and driving was dangerous. So I keep busy around the house, watching aging parents, and doing things to help wherever I can with family and friends. If I am busy doing yard work and chores around the house, the pain in my feet sometimes creeps back, and by the end of the day I am ready for sleep and grounding, but again in the morning I feel good and pain free.

"I can't express enough how much it has helped me in just feeling better overall. Behcet's did a job on my body and grounding has made my life better. I feel blessed, and I am happy to be alive."

ELECTROSENSITIVITY

"Electropollution" is slang for the unseen, unfelt, and unnatural EMFs, the electromagnetic fields generated by everything from high-tension electrical wires, wiring in the walls of homes and offices, and many appliances. Some people are highly sensitive—allergic, you might say— to EMF emissions. They can develop headaches, arthritic pain, insomnia, chest discomfort and heart arrhythmias, anxiety, and depression. EMF sensitivity is rarely diagnosed, and although these individuals may take medication, their symptoms rarely go away. Researchers in Europe suggest that 3 to 6 percent of the population is affected by EMF exposure.

Step Sinatra, whose story you will read next, is the eldest son of co-author Stephen Sinatra. Despite all the best care that Dr. Sinatra could arrange, he and his family watched anxiously while Step's health deteriorated over several years. "I don't really have to look very far to see the damage that electropollution can do," says Dr. Sinatra. "There was great fear we might lose Step. Doctors diagnosed him variously as having an autoimmune disorder, parasites, and even mercury toxicity. We now strongly believe that electropollution set him up for internal dysfunction and negatively affected his body's innate intelligence to heal itself. He has made a remarkable recovery, literally from death's door."

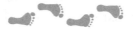

Step Sinatra, thirty-three, Encinitas, California, entrepreneur: "In the late 1990s, I was trading stocks on Wall Street, on a floor with a hundred guys surrounded by a battery of computers, phones, and electronics. I got my first cell phone in 1997 and another one a year later. I used them all the time. I worked in this intense environment from 9:00 a.m. to market closing time.

"I was in constant overdrive, filled with a zest for life and a desire to experience it all. I was young, strong, and healthy. I worked hard, took enormous risks, and felt I could handle it all. I was living the Manhattan lifestyle. I had an apartment on the forty-third floor that faced the World Trade Towers five blocks away.

"I didn't know it at the time, but I was being bombarded 24/7 by

EMFs and cell phone tower emissions. For the four years I worked on Wall Street I didn't sleep much. I was wired. In time, I began to feel something affecting my health. I thought it was the high stress level of my work. Then things started to go wrong. I developed ear, eye, and nose problems, a chronic cough, and major congestion. My symptoms got worse, but I didn't stop and listen. I felt I would get healthy later. I was making serious money and living an ego-driven, high stress lifestyle.

"However, at one point I had chest pains that my father thought might be coronary artery spasms or an early warning of a heart attack. I was twenty-five years old!

"The experience stopped me in my tracks. I realized I was really beaten down and was smart enough to know when to throw in the towel. In 2001, after the attack on the World Trade Towers, I moved to Colorado and worked on getting my health back. But I just kept deteriorating. I was starting to get scared.

"I set up a small office in Boulder—a trading operation—and filled it with wireless networks and cordless phones, not knowing the harm they were causing me. I worked and slept there, so I was getting hit with EMFs day and night. I still didn't understand what I had. All I knew was I was getting worse, with weight loss, weakness, severe bloating and gas, inability to digest certain foods, muscle pains, injuries, sleep issues, and food allergies.

"I became as tenacious about my health as I had been before trading stocks. I consulted with nutritionists, acupuncturists, far-out alternative therapists, and conventional doctor after doctor. My father was also trying to help me. I did blood test after inconclusive blood test. Nobody knew what was wrong. I kept fading away, losing two or three pounds a month no matter what I did.

"I had to get out of trading, but I still needed my laptop and cell phone because I worked for myself. I began to strongly suspect that EMFs were harmful because exposure made me feel worse. I don't know if I was always sensitive to EMFs or developed an extreme sensitivity on Wall Street.

"My father had me see some of the best doctors in the country he knew. Nobody could figure it out. I spent hundreds of thousands of dollars and read almost every book I could get my hands on, and still I got worse. I spent $20,000 of my own money at one famous clinic and they couldn't figure anything out. They just said I had endocrine problems. It was scary knowing that something was seriously wrong and yet no doctor knew why I got sick or why I was doing so poorly. Only one thing was clear in all the confusion: I became a defenseless host, vulnerable to heavy metals and any parasites that came along.

"I reached a culmination point in 2007 when I went to a clinic for a parasite infection. I spent three weeks on parasitic medicines and a raw food diet to help cleanse my body. However, I lost another thirty-five pounds in several weeks. My body completely shut down, and I had to be hospitalized. I was six feet tall and weighed eighty-three pounds. My liver, kidney, and blood tests were off the charts! And there I was in a hospital surrounded by a lot of electromagnetic monitoring devices and equipment. I couldn't eat or digest any food. I had to be fed via intravenous nutrition. That's what saved me, along with the prayers and love from family and friends.

"I was in the hospital for forty days. In the beginning, it looked like I wouldn't make it. The doctors gave me a 1 percent chance. If I did live, they had no idea what my life would be like because my body had eaten most of itself. I was in excruciating pain. I couldn't go to the bathroom because I was pretty much paralyzed. I was utterly vulnerable. There were times I was so weak that if a visitor walked into the room talking on a cell phone I would feel nauseous. If somebody brought a laptop to show me pictures, I couldn't look at it for more than a minute. I was that sensitive and had become increasingly aware of my sensitivity.

"One night I almost choked while taking a sip of water, and I thought I was gone. So did my dad, who was with me. But in that moment something Divine manifested, a sort of spiritual awakening or angelic intervention. I suddenly knew that we create our fears, dreams, and almost everything else. It was the worst and best moment of my life at the same time. I realized that with the intention of spirit I could create anything. I asked God for a miracle, and my prayer was answered. I felt reconnected and knew I would recover. I felt all I wanted to do was help people. This was my purpose and I had a message.

"I started to reverse course and improve. In the spring of 2008, I was strong enough to leave the hospital. I was still super fragile, though. My father talked to me around this time about Earthing, even just sitting with my bare feet on the grass. As the weather warmed up, I started sitting, standing, and walking barefoot a bit. I noticed my strength coming back slowly. I made sure that there were very few electromagnetic gadgets in my vicinity.

"Once, I had a big relapse when cordless phones and wireless Internet were set up in the room I was recovering in. I developed a *Salmonella* infection in my bladder and had to be hospitalized again. After that I obtained an electromagnetic detector that alerted me to the unseen EMFs harming me. I became extremely wary about my environment and cleared out any electrical and electronic stuff. I immediately felt and slept better. I didn't use a computer for the first nine months out of the hospital. I wouldn't even look at one. I stopped speaking on a cell phone unless absolutely necessary and that might be only once or twice a month. I only used a corded phone and a computer connected to a landline. No wireless.

"Shortly after I got out of the hospital, I started sleeping grounded. It was amazing. The first few nights, I got perhaps six or seven hours of sleep, but I woke up feeling better each day—compared to sleeping nine or ten hours previously and waking up feeling poorly. I felt such a dramatic boost in energy and health that I have not slept ungrounded since. When I travel, I take my grounding sheet with me. On one trip, I arrived at my hotel rather late and set up my sheet. I slept very poorly that night and realized the next morning I had forgotten to connect it. That was a big confirmation for me that Earthing was very effective and instrumental in my healing. I've actually been able to handle more EMFs as I got stronger. When I use a computer, I have my feet on a grounded floor mat, so I'm able to stay on the computer much longer than before. If I'm not grounded, after about ten minutes I get hot, sweaty, and uncomfortable.

"Today, at 150 pounds, I am stronger than I have been in years. I'm blessed to be alive. I pray that others become more aware of EMFs without having to endure the path that I did, and can live this wonderful gift of life to the fullest."

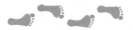

Edie Miller, fifty-six, Inman, South Carolina, bookkeeper: "Extreme sensitivity to electromagnetic fields keeps me from working outside my home. I literally feel the energy coming in to my body, and it is very disturbing. From 2000 to 2005, I was forced to leave three different jobs because of this sensitivity. After quitting I would have to recuperate at home. I didn't know what was causing the problems and was going to doctors for fixes, but they didn't understand what was happening either. I had to figure it out on my own and until I did my life seemed to be one health crisis after another.

"Sleeping became a big problem. It was as if all the cells in my body were vibrating. Over time, this sensation became more and more intense. The vibrating became faster and faster. I had no idea what it was. Later, I understood that it had to do with my sensitivity and probably the wiring in my house. This went on every night. Many times I wouldn't get to sleep until 3:00 or 4:00 a.m. There were nights I didn't sleep at all. I would get totally exhausted, and then I would sleep. Doctors couldn't help me. They wanted to give me sleeping pills, which wouldn't solve my problem. I lived in a constant state of sleep deprivation and chronic fatigue. If I sat down to watch television, I would fall asleep. My husband and I used to play tennis and cycle regularly. All that stopped. I am not a cranky or depressed person by nature, and I was becoming quite cranky, depressed, and unhappy. When you don't get enough sleep, everything bothers you. I had this problem for ten years.

"I also had physical problems. I had been a purchasing agent for one of the country's biggest suppliers of canvas, nylon, and other fabrics for commercial industrial, recreational and clothing applications. I worked at a computer all day. I was having major problems with my right shoulder as a result of using the mouse. The mouse put a wallop on me more than the keyboard. Just putting my hand on the mouse I could feel the energy going up my arm, and it was very uncomfortable. At first I thought I had pulled a tendon in my shoulder. One doctor wanted to perform rotator cuff surgery, but I was very scared to have it. My dad had had that surgery done and never had good use of his arm after that. I had bodywork done with the shoulder and it helped a lot.

"I had lots of problems picking up things. At another job, I worked as a cashier. By the end of the day, the muscles in my right arm had no strength at all. That was the hand that I used to work the register. Just picking up a loaf of bread was difficult. I felt the electrical energy coming into me through the register.

"In an effort to get away from working with registers, computers, or anything electronic, I got a job at one of the big chain bookstores stocking books. I worked there for two years. In the beginning I was okay, but increasingly we were working with battery-operated electronic scanners. While using this device I developed trigger finger, a painful condition in which fingers or thumbs lock up in a bent position. You can straighten them out with a snap. Women develop this more than men, and I was one. Both my thumbs were affected, along with my right index and middle finger and left index finger. I went to a doctor, but the treatment did nothing for the condition. I also developed tennis elbow. In fact, every joint on the right side of my body was affected, including my right knee. I got to the point where I couldn't even lift the books up to the shelf or raise myself after squatting down to place books on a bottom shelf. I am very small and it had nothing to do with weight.

"I learned about Earthing on the Internet in 2004. This seemed like something that might help me deal with my problem. I sure needed something. I got myself a grounded floor pad and put it in my bed, so that my feet rested on it. I felt the difference immediately—the very first night. The cells in my body just stopped vibrating. The night before I had a typical night of maybe three or four hours of sleep. With the pad, I fell asleep right away. I woke up at 9:30 or 10:00 a.m. feeling a sense of blessed relief. For about three months I would sleep late like that, something I had never done before. My body was apparently catching up with lost sleep. Then my sleep simply normalized. When 7:00 a.m. comes, I'm up and ready to go. My depression faded away and my energy picked up. I was able to exercise regularly again. The trigger fingers started loosening up within a week of sleeping grounded, and in about a month, they were 100 percent functional.

"Needless to say, I sleep grounded all the time. I work at the computer at home and use another floor pad at my desk. I can work all day, even with a mouse, without any problem as long as I am grounded. I take a pad with me when we travel. If I don't, the problem comes right back and immediately. I still have my electrosensitivity, and I am reminded of it every day, but I can live with it and function pretty normally as long as I stay grounded."

FIBROMYALGIA

Fibromyalgia is a common chronic pain condition affecting an estimated 3 to 6 percent of the world population, including 10 million Americans, more than three-quarters of whom are women. According to the National Fibromyalgia Association, the causes "still remain a mystery." The primary symptom is chronic widespread body pain, along with moderate to extreme fatigue and sleep disturbances. Often there are overlapping conditions, such as irritable bowel, lupus, and arthritis.

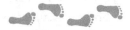

Armida Champagne, sixty-eight, San Diego, real estate agent: "In 1995, I was diagnosed with fibromyalgia. That, along with arthritis, was making my life increasingly miserable. I had a very hard time sleeping because of the pain. Just lying in bed hurt, and on top of that, I couldn't sit too long in any one place either. I wasn't disabled to the point where I couldn't do things, but I was in a lot of pain. And I was tired all the time. The pain was always there, and in the evening it was particularly bad. On a scale of 1 to 10, the pain was probably at an 8 level every night. The pain was all over, from my shoulders down to my toes. It would often wake me up.

"I tried all kinds of remedies, creams, and pain relievers. They might help for about an hour or so but that was it. I avoided taking any strong painkillers, but on occasion I would use Aleve, a non-steroidal anti-inflammatory over-the-counter medication, and that would help me for a while longer.

"In 2000, I started grounding myself at night with one of the first prototype bed pads. The very first night, I fell asleep right away and woke up refreshed without any pain. I couldn't believe it. The pain was completely gone. To be sure, I have slept grounded ever since. I also have a pad on my couch, so when I lie down to relax or watch TV I am getting in some extra grounding time.

"Every once and awhile I get a twinge of pain but never like it was before. I sleep for eight hours straight. Sometimes for nine or ten. I feel fantastic and with plenty of energy. I don't know how I would be without this pad, especially with all the stress involved in my real estate work the last few years.

"Occasionally, I visit a cousin in Santa Barbara and I bring my bed pad with me. The first time I brought it, I plugged it into what I thought was a grounded wall outlet in the guest bedroom. But I didn't sleep well that night or the next. I also started to hurt a bit. I asked my cousin about the electrical system in the house. She said the bedroom wasn't grounded, but the kitchen and bathrooms were. So I took an extension cord with a ground prong and plugged it into an outlet in the kitchen, which was grounded. I immediately felt the difference that night and slept well.

"I was also amazed at the effect of sleeping grounded on my significant other. He had a slight sleep apnea problem diagnosed by his doctor. He used to wake up during the night, gasping for breath. Sometimes he could go back to sleep right away. Other times not. He also used to snore so loud that I couldn't go to sleep. I would have to go to bed first and then he would come in later. The grounding changed all that as well. In a couple of months, his snoring tapered off and then stopped. The apnea took longer but it also eased up and then went away. He hasn't had that problem for more than four years.

"For the last five years of her life, my mother slept grounded. She died in 2005 at the age of ninety-six. She was a horrible snorer until she slept grounded. Her snoring stopped as well, and I believe the grounding gave her some comfort and ease in those last years of her life."

JET LAG

Jim Bagnola, sixty, Austin, Texas, leadership consultant and corporate educator: "In my work, I travel all over the world, so jet lag is always an issue. In my experience, going barefoot and sleeping grounded are the fastest ways to realign to a far-flung time zone. I also sleep more soundly, with more lucid dreaming, and feel stronger physically.

"In the past I have tried all kinds of treatments, remedies, and gadgets to counteract jet lag. Walking on grass and sleeping grounded works for me the most effectively. After returning home to Texas from a recent trip to France, England, and Romania, I recovered within a couple of days. It would otherwise take me a week after an extended trip like that.

"When I arrive at foreign destinations and check into my hotel, I walk barefoot on grass wherever I can find it. This has been a hilarious experience at times. I travel to Romania quite a bit, and in downtown Bucharest I take advantage of a good patch of grass in front of the National Theatre, next door to the Intercontinental Hotel. As I do my twenty minutes of barefoot walking there, people will often stop and watch me circling the grassy area in my bare feet. Some ask what I am doing. I attempt to tell them about grounding and jet lag, and they look at me as if I am crazy. Many cannot speak English so it makes the situation rather humorous. I did get a bee sting once so I have to be careful where I walk. But otherwise it works great."

MIXED CONNECTIVE TISSUE DISEASE

Mixed connective tissue disease (MCTD) is an autoimmune disorder sometimes called an overlap disease because it manifests with signs and symptoms of several other connective tissue diseases: lupus, scleroderma, and polymyositis. This condition occurs mostly in women. Symptoms may include fatigue, muscle weakness, joint pain and swelling, and difficulty swallowing. Many patients have difficulty breathing as a result of inflammation of the lining that covers the lungs and the inside of the chest.

Lynne Corwin, sixty-three, Hemet, California: "Ten years ago I became very ill. After many tests, the doctors diagnosed mixed connective tissue disease. The condition stopped me in my tracks. The doctors said the statistics indicated I had three years to live. They recommended I go home, get my affairs in order, and whenever I had a good day I should enjoy it. The implication was clear that there wouldn't be too many good days. They essentially wrote me off.

"For years, I was in a very bad way, just sitting painfully on the sidelines and watching the world go by. I went from one prescription to another. I couldn't be the active grandmother that I wanted to be for my five grandchildren.

"At some particularly low point, I decided I had to try to lift myself up by my bootstraps and do whatever I could to improve my quality of life. I recall that one day between breakfast and lunch I resolved to become a strict vegetarian and stay away from fatty and processed foods. That made a difference. Later I met Richard Delany, a medical doctor who integrates conventional and alternative medicine in his practice. He has helped me a great deal. In March of 2009, he recommended I sleep grounded as part of his evolving therapeutic strategy. In the six months since that time, I have slept ungrounded only one night. I take the grounded sleeping bag with me whenever I travel.

"It is hard to pinpoint the specific improvements from any individual treatments I have received. But ever since I started sleeping grounded, there has been noticeable improvement all around, and certainly with my primary symptoms of shortness of breath and difficulty swallowing.

"I haven't had problems sleeping in the past. What has changed is the quality of sleep. I noticed it the very first night I slept grounded. Profoundly restful is the best way I can describe it. It was the same the next night and the night after that, and it has continued. After a while, I guess I became accustomed to this wonderful quality of sleep.

"One of my problems is reflux if I lie flat, so I have to sleep on an incline or in a chair, sitting up. This is because my esophagus has deteriorated. It doesn't work right. It doesn't retain contents in my stomach if, for instance, I bend over. The content may come right up, and when it does, I have tremendous pain in the throat and my ears will hurt. I have been taking extremely high doses of acid suppressants for years to counteract this problem. Thanks to Dr. Delany's guidance, I have been able to significantly decrease the dosage, and dramatically so since I've slept grounded. We have eliminated one medication altogether at night and cut back on another by two-thirds. Needless to say, I am very excited about this.

In the past, when I felt poorly I couldn't think straight. There was mental confusion and I was in the doldrums. Since grounding myself I have found my brain operates clearer. My thinking processes are more precise. Despite not being able to function the way I would like, I seem to be more cheerful than before. And I also have more energy than before. Prior to being grounded I couldn't get through the day without an afternoon nap, anywhere from a half hour to two hours. Now I don't need to nap at all. That's how improved I am.

"There was a time when I couldn't read a story to my grandkids. I didn't have the breath to do it. Breathlessness is still a problem, but now it's less of a problem and I can get through a story with perhaps just a momentary rest or two."

MULTIPLE SCLEROSIS

Multiple sclerosis (MS) is a degenerative disease of the central nervous system that typically emerges in young adults and can lead to severe disability. Symptoms often include aching, loss of balance, muscle spasms, paralysis, and general fatigue. Experts roughly estimate that 1.3 million individuals globally are affected, but many regard that number as a "big underestimation." As least twice as many women as men are affected. The highest incidence of MS occurs in countries the farthest away from the Equator, and experts believe this is possibly due to less sunlight, environmental factors, or dietary reasons. Among the unrecognized environmental factors is lack of grounding. Our observations are that when patients with MS are grounded, they get better.

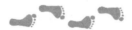

Cindy Walsh, forty-seven, Southern California marriage and family therapist: "I was diagnosed with multiple sclerosis in 1999 at a time when there was a lot of stress in my life. The symptoms included a sensation of heaviness throughout my left side that would last for thirty seconds or so. My right hand would twist up, so that my palm faced upward. I was prescribed three medications, but I dropped them after six weeks because of the side effects. One of them, an injectable, gave me fevers, chills, and achiness. A year after my diagnosis I had to go on disability. I had limited amounts of energy and had to carefully balance my schedule around my two beautiful and active young children and the need for rest.

"I had several years where things were fairly good. I was exercising a lot, swimming, and even walking for miles. It was great. But in 2007 I had a bad flare-up. My rib cage would tighten, as if a girdle was tightly squeezing me. It was very uncomfortable. My whole body felt strange.

"In 2008, it was record-breaking hot where I live, and heat is an enemy for someone with MS. I had the worst flare I've ever had. It was very scary. My left arm stopped working, as if it was no longer connected to my brain. It would move on its own and I couldn't grip anything. I couldn't type with my left hand. My arm just became useless. And then my legs started feeling strange.

"It was around this time that a friend told me about a study being conducted nearby on something called Earthing. The friend thought that maybe this could help me. I found out that participants had to sit for a period of time while the testing was going on, and I wasn't sure I could last that long. Still, I was invited to come over anyway one weekend when the study wasn't going on, just to see if Earthing could help my condition.

"That's when I met Clint Ober. He hooked me up, and I sat there for a while. It felt very soothing and I enjoyed it. When I was unhooked, I got up and went to the restroom. In the restroom I took one look at myself in the mirror and couldn't believe what I saw. It was as if I had slept for three days or been on a healing retreat. I looked so much better and younger. I'd been very tired, sad, and stressed out. I was amazed.

"Clint gave me some grounding paraphernalia to take home and try out. I've been sleeping grounded most of the time ever since. Despite going through a very stressful year, including surgery, the grounding gives me a genuine sense of comfort. I haven't had a flare since starting, despite all the stress. And my energy level is up. I'm looking at my body, and I'm thinking about what I've been through and how well I'm doing.

"I just passed my tenth anniversary of being diagnosed with MS. I got through the last flare in a really beautiful way. For several years, some dear friends have helped me get hyperbaric oxygen treatments. I eat a good diet with as much organic food as possible. I take B vitamin shots. I have been doing a lot of things for my health, and then I added Earthing. It's part of my 'healing team.' I do believe it makes a big difference and has helped keep me feeling the way I do. I sit on the grounding sheet sometimes while reading or watching movies. I make sure I do more than just sleep on it. I'm actually doing really, really well."

SCIATICA

Sciatica refers to leg pain caused by compression of the nerves coming out of the lower spine and forming the major nerve in the leg, the sciatic nerve. There may also be pain in the low back and buttock, along with tingling and numbness in the lower extremities.

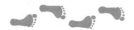

Mike Miller, sixty-two, Encinitas, California, retired software engineer: "I have had sciatica since 1966—over forty years. I pulverized my fourth, fifth, and sixth lumbar vertebrae in a car accident and have lived with a great deal of pain and discomfort ever since. There is nothing medically that can be done about the situation except to take aspirin, which relieves the swelling of the sciatic nerve where it exits the spine. Aspirin actually works pretty well, but not perfectly. It does not eliminate the pain but relieves the swelling, which reduces the pain to a manageable level. For forty-two years I have basically taken two aspirin every night.

"My symptoms were extremely painful shooting pains usually down my right leg to the knee and sometimes all the way to the middle of the foot, which contracts like a fist. I say usually because, in some cases, it would switch to the left leg and on really bad nights affect both legs. Additionally, I was dealing with a constant low-grade pain in the lower back, the muscles around the knees, back of the thighs, and the calves of both legs. The pain was there every night. It exhausted me. I usually took about an hour to an hour and a half to fall asleep. And when I did finally fall asleep, it was from exhaustion. When I woke up, I usually felt like I had jet lag or a hangover.

"In early 2008, I started sleeping grounded and everything changed. I experienced an immediate cessation of all the symptoms. I was stunned. I couldn't get over it. I just laid down and went right to sleep without a sciatic attack. I woke up the next day and said, 'Hey, I slept all night!' That was the first time I slept through the night in five years. I didn't have to go through my nightly ritual of discomfort before falling off to sleep. From the very beginning, I knew this was something special.

"I have been using the pad every night since, plugged into my wall socket. I even took the pad camping and used a grounding rod with it and could sleep in our camper without the least discomfort! That's a first too.

"In general I have no symptoms or pain, or need for medication, as long as I behave myself. By that I mean not lifting something too heavy or otherwise overdoing it, which, unfortunately I do from time to time. I'll irritate the nerve and have to take three aspirins to cut the pain. The next day, though, I am okay again.

"The results have been remarkable. I couldn't do much for years, and any kind of stress would aggravate my condition. I wasn't able to garden for four years. Now, I'm able to garden again and do light physical work. I can handle stress much better. I have my life back again."

Better Sleep

Nearly everybody who sleeps grounded says they sleep better, including globe-trotting celebrities.

Actor Orlando Bloom: "It's the best sleep."

Chad Reed, World Supercross Champion: "No matter the work load I put on my body, I'm recovered for the next day when I sleep grounded."

Supermodel Miranda Kerr: "Sleeping grounded gives me sound uninterrupted sleep. I awake feeling refreshed, even with all my traveling."

SLEEP APNEA

An estimated 20 million Americans have sleep apnea. This means episodes of impaired breathing and disturbed sleep caused by a narrowing of soft tissue in the upper airway. Apnea reduces oxygen in the blood and prompts arousal from sleep. A continuous positive airway pressure (CPAP) machine is widely used as a remedy. It delivers a stream of compressed air via a hose to a nasal pillow, nose mask, or full-face mask. The pressure keeps the airway open. Researchers think that obstructive sleep apnea activates an inflammatory response in the body that may contribute to cardiovascular disease.

Daryl James, eighty-three, Palm Springs, California, business consultant and writer: "Increasingly, over a period of a few years, I would wake up a few times a night gasping for breath. Finally, I went to a sleep clinic. The tests indicated that I had a moderate case of sleep apnea, with episodes where I would stop breathing for twenty seconds at a time. A lot of sleep apnea patients die in their sleep. I didn't want to be one of them.

"I was told to get a CPAP machine. I did just that. I used it every night and it helped me sleep without interruption, but I didn't like using the device. It's not very comfortable.

"After hearing about grounding and how it improved sleep, I decided to give it a try it and see if it could possibly help my situation. It did!

"There were times when the CPAP face mask was too uncomfortable so I removed it. And even without it, I was able to get through the night without any problem. I noticed this within a few months of grounding. Now, I've been sleeping grounded for about almost a year and hardly ever need to use the CPAP anymore. I've been able to wean myself off. I had a serious condition, and there is no doubt the grounding helped me cope and recover.

"As a result, I have found that I have more energy during the day. In addition, my blood pressure has stabilized. I have been on hypertensive medication, but the blood pressure control hasn't been as good as my doctor would like to see it. I've been able to noticeably control the pressure better since being grounded."

STRESS RELIEF

Scott Hyatt, forty-five, Northern California law enforcement officer: "I work in narcotics, and my life can be very stressful from just the people I come in contact with, to making time for court, and for family and everything else. In my work, I can be one minute on surveillance, sitting there and nothing's happening. And the next minute, I'm out of the car and running, trying to get my raid vest on and my weapon out. So the stresses are from zero up to 100 miles an hour at any given time.

"Sleep takes a hit in all this irregularity. My sleep routine was skewed at best. So there's a lot of fatigue. In my job I've broken my foot, my hand, my nose, and my wrist. So there are also aches and pains from that, as well as a stiff back from wearing gun belts and raid vests.

"I've been sleeping grounded for about six years. And it made a huge difference. I used to be up a lot in the middle of the night—tossing and turning, fluffing my pillow, getting up, stretching, getting back into bed. And after I started using the bed pad, I've been getting a better quality of sleep—maybe not as much time as I would like because we still have strange hours we have to work with, but the quality of sleep really improved.

"There's also been a big difference in the aches and pains. They're gone. I didn't even really notice it until after six months or so. I woke up one morning and got right out of bed and there were no aches and pains, no sore back, no sore feet. It was amazing. I had probably not had any pain or stiffness before that but hadn't noticed it.

"I'm an avid runner, and so I'm used to the aches and pains of my ankles, knees, and hip flexors. They were gone as well. When I was out running later that day, it just kept reoccurring to me that something had changed and it wasn't my job, it wasn't my eating habits, it wasn't anything else. I could only put it to the bed pad.

"When I would run races—like five kilometers—and trying to beat my friends I would be running faster than when I'm out just on my own. The next morning I would usually be plenty sore and achy. The bed pad has taken that away as well. The aches are minimal. It's amazing."

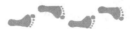

Brad Graham, fifty-four, Lakewood, California, firefighter: "This job, as you can imagine, involves a lot of stress, physically and mentally. You never know what you are going to face at any particular time of the day or night.

"You could be asleep at 1:00 a.m., and you get a call. It may be to respond to a fire or to a situation where people are trapped in a car that's been in an accident. You go from deep rest to fast and furious action and saving lives.

"When you get back to the station, it's hard to get the scenes of what you have been through out of your mind. If you rescue somebody who was injured, you wonder if they will be okay. And you may think about what you could have done different to affect the outcome.

"Because of the nature of the work, sometimes it is very, very difficult to get back to sleep after a call. Sometimes I'll lie in bed for hours. Sometimes I'll even get up, take a shower, and go to the kitchen and read the paper.

"When I sleep grounded, I find I am able to go back to sleep after a call in what I would consider a decent time period. Maybe twenty minutes versus two and a half hours. I also notice that I sleep deeper and feel more rested when I get up in the morning. I'm more rested, but still alert.

"There seems to be a physical benefit as well. Our type of work can be quite strenuous. I think some of the issues that firefighters face, especially as the years take their toll on us, is that our knees get a little stiff. Or, as we get older, we develop back problems. Ever since I've been sleeping grounded, my knees don't feel as stiff as they used to. I like to maintain my strength by lifting weights. For quite a while, I pretty much wasn't able to do squats. Now, at the gym, I can perform squats again. And I'm able to run better than before."

VARICOSE VEINS AND BAD CIRCULATION

Roland Perez, sixty-six, Palm Desert, California, medical film producer: "Experts say that some people are likely to inherit varicose veins, and I appear to be one of them. My mother had a severe case, and so did I. It left my feet, up to the ankles, almost black in some places, particularly on the instep. The veins were getting smaller and the circulation was not very good. My feet were very cold, and as I walked around, I didn't have much feeling in them. I could walk on cold tile and not feel the cold. I didn't know what to do about it. There was nothing that doctors could do for it.

"Then I heard about Earthing and got a grounded bed pad. It was a Sunday afternoon when I first tried it out. I lay there for about twenty minutes, watching television. There had been no pain before. Now there was bad pain. The feet started to spasm. I jumped up and said, 'Done, I'm not doing this.'

"The next day I spoke to Clint Ober and told him about the pain. He suggested that what I had experienced was not uncommon and was very likely part of an initial healing response. So I decided to continue. Within two days the pain went away. It was replaced by tingling in my feet for about three weeks. Then I started noticing that the color in my feet was getting lighter. I thought to myself that this couldn't be possible. It is not something that you could clear up. But it was clearing up.

"Before my feet used to get very dry, crack, and sometimes bleed. I would develop sores. All a result of bad circulation. Slowly, my feet softened on the bottom. The cracking and bleeding stopped.

"These improvements happened within two months. I hadn't said anything to my wife. One day during breakfast, she noticed my feet. She was surprised. 'Your feet really look good,' she said.

"By five months, the color of my feet had cleared up completely. Both feet.

"My wife has varicose veins on the back of her legs, and she used to put makeup on the back of her legs. She wondered if grounding would help her. After six weeks, one leg was totally clear. The other has a slight purplish curved line. The legs have definitely have improved. We haven't done anything other than be grounded."

THE YOGIS KNEW

John Gray, fifty-eight, Mill Valley California, author of *Men Are from Mars, Women Are from Venus* (Harper Collins, 1992): "The concept of Earthing resonates deeply with me. I have, in fact, done something similar since 1995 when I was in India and studying with teachers of the Indian meditation system. It was recommended to me that for the best results in my practice I should sleep and meditate on a deerskin, and the deerskin should be on the ground.

"This was the tradition of the Yogis. The teachers said there was energy from above that comes to the Earth and then comes to you if you stay connected to the Earth. The Yogis, of course, would meditate for long periods of time and always do so on an animal skin. They often lived in caves where they would be surrounded by the Earth. They would also put down little sheets and sleep on earthen or marble floors as well. The Christian mystics had practices like this. They would go out into the desert and meditate in Nature, knowing that the results were better.

"When I was in India, I wasn't very interested in sleeping on the ground. The Yogis said there was another option for me, something that the kings did when they studied Yogic techniques in the past and apparently received benefits in terms of longer life. The option was the use of a bed sheet made with copper material that was connected to a copper rod outside, placed in the ground. I guess they did a lot with metal thousands of years ago. They certainly had some specific knowledge.

"I obtained a setup like this in India and used it in my home. At the time, I had some pain from bursitis in the shoulder. I'd had it for two or three years. I would feel it particularly when I woke up. Then, after sleeping on the Indian sheets for a while, the pains were not there anymore.

"I had the Indian sheets for about twelve years and enjoyed them very much. Then I moved the bed and the original wire wouldn't reach so I stopped using the copper sheets for a while. Then I heard of Clint Ober's work and obtained some conductive sheets that he had developed. One of the first things I noticed is that I could no longer sleep later than 8:00 a.m. Even if I am up late the night before, there's no way I can sleep past 8:00 a.m. Yet I am up at that time, fully refreshed. That's part of normalizing the circadian rhythm. Your cortisol level is highest at that time. There's no possibility anymore of sleeping late for me when I'm on those sheets.

"Other people who I have turned on to Earthing have had positive experiences. I've heard about arthritic pains going away in a few days and restless legs immediately calming down."

Keep Track of Your Earthing Experience

To monitor how Earthing may be helping you, we have created a simple symptom checklist and progress chart. You'll find it in Appendix D.

CHAPTER 11

The Heart Connection: Steve Sinatra's Perspective

Earthing research is in its bare infancy as far as the heart and cardiology is concerned. Yet our observations and the feedback from patients point to an exciting potential: an utterly simple method that can both protect healthy hearts and help heal ailing ones. In addition, we can perhaps draw some assurance at this early date in our research knowing that countless barefoot and much-closer-to-Nature generations that came before us were pretty much free of heart disease. Today, it is the No. 1 disease killer in the Western world and is rising rapidly in tropical and subtropical countries where it was previously uncommon. As a cardiologist who uses both conventional and complementary methods, I envision Earthing becoming a major practical tool against cardiovascular disease. In fact, it looks like a big winner in the practice of medicine in general.

Like any new idea in the medical world, Earthing needs to be carefully scrutinized and tested objectively without bias. If that happens, I see it taking a central place as a natural, low-cost pillar of health maintenance and disease prevention and treatment. In this age of off-the-chart medical costs and skyrocketing chronic disease, doctors need as much help as we can get in order to give patients cost-effective care. Where better to get that help than from Mother Earth herself? From the ground up, no less.

I am excited by the broad implications of key improvements related to the following:

- ATP production

- Sympathetic nervous system activity

- Arrhythmias

- High blood pressure

- Blood viscosity

With time, I am confident that many more benefits will come to light. Meantime, I'd like to discuss what we know now about Earthing and its positive effects on the heart and cardiovascular system.

PROMOTING THE BODY'S ENERGY FUEL—ATP

For me, a metabolic cardiologist keenly interested in improving and maintaining the energy production in the hearts and bodies of patients, Earthing has all the makings of a simple, safe, and effective energy booster. For years, I have recommended natural supplements such as coenzyme Q10 (CoQ10), L-carnitine, D-ribose, and magnesium to elevate the bioenergetics of nutrient-starved heart cells and protect them from the ravages of aging, environmental toxins, and relentless oxidation. I have written books and articles about these supplements I refer to as "the awesome foursome." They provide key metabolic raw materials that are typically deficient in patients. This nutritional approach has worked remarkably and consistently well in helping to restore the failing pumping capacity of sick hearts. Now, Earthing appears to provide another primary ingredient for cellular restoration and cardiac rehabilitation.

The Earth feeds energy into all organisms that make direct contact with it. One aspect of this bioelectrical energizing likely takes place in the mitochondria of your trillions of cells. The mitochondria are like microscopic power plants. There can be thousands of them in each cell, depending on how much energy the cell has to provide (heart and kidney cells contain the most). Inside the mitochondria, a complex process takes place nonstop. In it, electrons are passed along, like a football, through an assembly line of enzymes that create a substance called adenosine triphosphate (ATP), the fuel that enables cells to function and repair themselves. By providing an unlimited flow of electrons into the body, grounding may ensure that ample electrons are available in the mitochondria and may thus contribute to the production of ATP in all the cells.

It's taken me the better part of thirty-five years of practicing cardiology to learn that the heart is all about ATP. The bottom line in the treatment of any form of cardiovascular disease is the restoration of your heart's supply of ATP. I've come to realize that sick hearts leak out and lose vital ATP. Cardiac conditions such as angina, heart failure, silent ischemia, and diastolic dysfunction can all cause an ATP deficit.

Another aspect of cellular energy production is that the electrons transported through the assembly line are of a higher energy type, more like a "hot potato" than a football, and that this energy is transferred to ATP. Scientists say these energized electrons are in an "excited state." We think that electrons provided by the Earth must be of that type—electrons brimming with higher energy. The Earth thus provides us not only more electrons but supercharged electrons at that!

THE SYMPATHETIC-HRV CONNECTION

Whenever you can turn down the volume on stress in the body, it's good for the heart and that's one of the big benefits of Earthing.

Chronic stress triggers an excess release of the stress hormones, like cortisol and adrenaline. It also throws off the balance between the sympathetic nervous system and the parasympathetic nervous system. Too much sympathetic "arousal"—from stress—leads to the well-known fight-or-flight mode, an alert and readiness state that humans automatically switch on in reaction to an imminent danger, like fighting in a battle. In today's world, unpredictable social, financial, and political events conspire to keep stress levels at an unhealthy high level. More and more people live day to day in a state of physiological arousal. (Refer to the inset on page 166 for a list of factors that rev up the sympathetic nervous system.)

Revved-up sympathetic activity overwhelms the calming influence of the parasympathetic nervous system. The result, among other things, is a heightened risk of hypertension, arrhythmias, and even sudden death. One major yardstick of sympathetic overdrive is disturbance to what cardiologists call heart rate variability (HRV), a measurement of nervous system balance on heart function as well as an important indicator for both acute and chronic stress produced by mental load, anxiety, and emotional trauma. HRV refers to the beat-to-beat alterations in heart rate. People with

Factors Contributing to Sympathetic Nervous System Activation

Environmental and/or medical conditions

Air pollution (particulate matter <10 microns)

Congestive heart failure

Depression, anxiety

Hypertension

Insulin resistance, diabetes, or metabolic syndrome

Obesity

Sleep apnea

Psychosocial and behavioral conditions

Abuse of stimulants

Chronic stress

Hostility, anger, or rage

Sedentary lifestyle

Sleep deprivation

Smoking

Social isolation and loneliness

Sugar-laden diet

Pharmaceutical drugs

Beta-agonist bronchodilators

Peripheral alpha blockers

Short-acting calcium channel blockers

low variability are less able to "go with the flow" when faced with stress and are more prone to stress-related disorders, including cardiovascular disease.

In 2008, I participated with electrophysiologist Gaetan Chevalier, Ph.D., in an experiment to measure the effect of Earthing on HRV. We believe that the autonomic nervous system (ANS) is one, and possibly the first, of the major body systems to react to Earthing. The ANS serves the body as a rapid response mechanism to control a wide range of functions. Cardiovascular, respiratory, gastrointestinal, hormonal, urinary, and other systems are regulated by the ANS's sympathetic and parasympathetic branches.

Previous experiments have shown that grounded individuals experience a reduction in stress and a normalizing, balancing effect on ANS function.

In this new study, which will be published in 2010, data from twenty-eight healthy men and women (average age of forty-eight) showed that Earthing produces a trend toward improvement in HRV. Each participant was measured for forty minutes, grounded as well as ungrounded. The results give yet more strong evidence indicating its potential for balancing the nervous system and supporting cardiovascular health.

This represents an important finding. If there is a trend in forty minutes, what will sleeping grounded for six or eight hours do? Whenever there is an improvement in HRV, a reduction in sympathetic intensity and a better balance of the ANS takes place. The study gives us a glimpse of significant cardiac possibilities inviting more investigation. It hints at a cardiac-protective feature of Nature hitherto unknown. In our opinion, Earthing should be added to a host of other simple, cost-effective and non-invasive interventions that positively impact the ANS (for a list of these interventions, see the inset on page 168).

ARRHYTHMIAS AND EARTHING

Arrhythmias—whether of the skipped heartbeat variety or atrial fibrillation or malignant ventricular irregularities—are frequently set off by emotional stress and turmoil, situations that generate heightened sympathetic activity. Worry and fear can trigger these cardiovascular events. There is definitely a heart-brain "hotline."

Imagine living with a heart that vibrates, quivers, and races rapidly and erratically instead of beating in a steady, comfortable, and predictable rhythm. Atrial fibrillation is the medical name for this condition, the most common arrhythmia of the heart. Every year, 2 million or so people are diagnosed with "atrial fib" or "a-fib," as it is called for short. Although it isn't by itself life threatening, it can lead to heart failure or stroke. For sure, it can scare the heck out of most anybody who has it and drain his or her energy. People frequently think they are having a heart attack.

A-fib means there is an electrical problem in the heart. In a normal heart rhythm, the upper chambers of the heart—the atria—contract in unison in response to an electrical signal generated by pockets of specialized cardiac cells called the sinus node. In patients with a-fib, however, the conduction is deranged and electrical signals are scattered throughout the

Interventions to Improve Autonomic Nervous System Function

EARTHING

Lifestyle modifications

Exercise

Meditation, yoga, tai chi, qigong

Religiosity or faith

Restoration of normal sleep

Smoking cessation

Social support

Stress reduction, biofeedback

Weight loss

Medications

Angiotensin-converting enzyme
    (ACE) inhibitors

Beta blockers

Natural supplements

Omega-3 fatty acids

atria. Instead of contracting, the atria beat quickly and irregularly. This results in the loss of normal, synchronous pulsation and raises the risk of blood pooling inside the chambers, where it can form clots. Coumadin is usually prescribed to prevent clot formation.

Emergency interventions include electrical cardioversion to "break" the atria from fibrillating and allow the heart to resynchronize and reestablish control. This procedure involves a perfectly timed, low dose of electricity to give the conduction system a "jolt," which enables it to reset itself.

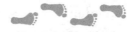

Bob Malone, sixty-nine, Boulder, Colorado, financial adviser: "After experiencing chest pain, rapid heart beat, and flutter, I was diagnosed with a-fib in 1996. It's very scary. You don't know when the next episode is going to come on and whether or not you will survive it. In my case, it was all brought on by stress in my life, particularly business stress. My work involves advice and decisions that affect people's lives.

"Medication kept the symptoms under control most of the time. When the meds were unable to control the wildness in my heart, I would have to get the electroshock and jolt the heart back into a normal rhythm. I needed that kind of treatment about every nine months or so. The meds were horrible. They took my energy down to zero. It was sort of like not having a life. I've always been an active, creative guy, and I love the outdoors, and now this stopped me in my tracks.

"I started sleeping grounded in 2000. I went from not getting sleep and waking up frequently at night to getting good, solid sleep pretty much all the time. I later added a grounded floor pad while I was reading or watching TV, and during the last couple of years, I have even used one at the office where the stress level is pretty high. I wear leather shoes so I can get the Earth's energy while I work.

"The number of incidents slowly started to stretch out. They went from days to weeks to months apart. Over time I was slowly able to wean myself off the medication. I had a flare-up in 2006, which I believe was related to the stress over the death of my brother. I had to take medication, but I haven't taken any for the last eighteen months.

"In 2007, I went to Vail for some fresh air and took an hour-and-a-half hike up and down a mountain. My pulse was ranging between 115 to 130 beats per minute. In the process I got chest pain (angina), which happens whenever I exercise aggressively. Then it normally goes away at night when I sleep grounded. But I wasn't grounded up in Vail, and the chest pain continued the following two days when I took two small hikes. I came back home the next day, a Sunday afternoon, with the pain still there. So I lay down on a grounded bed pad and napped for about a half hour. When I got up, the chest pain was gone completely. I even took a one-hour moderate bike ride afterward and no chest pain came back. So after having chest pain for three days straight I was greatly relieved.

"I haven't had chest pain since that time or any sign of atrial fib since October of 2008, about the time that the financial markets went sour. Despite all the stress that followed I didn't have another episode. Obviously I'm thrilled to have gone through the tough and anxious times without incident."

HIGH BLOOD PRESSURE

Doctors don't know the precise cause of high blood pressure, but they do know that it affects a huge segment of the human race and is increasing at an alarming rate. A 2007 report from health organizations around the world predicted a 60 percent rise, to an estimated 1.56 billion people by 2025. Currently, one billion people globally and about 72 million Americans have high blood pressure. The report envisioned a cardiovascular disease epidemic as a result. High blood pressure, while it is often symptomless, is serious business because it places you at increased risk for blindness, kidney damage, an enlarged heart, heart attack, and stroke.

High blood pressure is one of the biggest and most insidious heart risk factors around. Unless you get it under control, it is a sure ticket to heart disease. I've treated this common condition countless times in my practice and even wrote a book about it: *Lower Your Blood Pressure in Eight Weeks* (Ballantine, 2003).

I've often treated patients who came to me from other doctors unable to bring their blood pressure numbers down with conventional treatment. My experience has been that standard drug and diet therapies frequently fall far short of their intended goals, permitting incompletely controlled blood pressure to silently continue chipping away bits and pieces of the arterial system.

For a large percentage of patients with high blood pressure, I have used four major tools in a nondrug approach and they work both for prevention and therapy: diet, supplements, mind/body techniques, and exercise. Mild high blood pressure, as a matter of fact, is one of the easiest medical conditions to control without drugs or medical treatment. Management of emotional stress, optimal nutrition and supplements, weight management, exercise, elimination of smoking and caffeine, and moderate restriction of alcohol, as well as other lifestyle modifications can prevent, delay the onset, reduce the severity, treat and control the condition in many cases. Individuals with symptomatic kidney disease, a result of high blood pressure, need to take medication.

When I was in medical school more than thirty years ago, we didn't have a cause for high blood pressure. Now we regard the biggest cause as oxidative stress, meaning you have inflammation and free radicals eroding the sensitive endothelial cell linings of blood vessels. The second, and perhaps equally as big, is sympathetic overdrive that, among other things, causes the blood vessels to constrict.

As far as Earthing is concerned, we haven't done a study yet to document the effects on blood pressure, but our observations so far are very promising. Earthing snuffs out harmful free-radical activity and inflammation. It pacifies sympathetic overdrive. We think Earthing may represent the easiest possible way to lower your blood pressure. You do it in your sleep without a pill or anything else.

The following two stories show the possibilities.

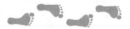

Dean W. Levin, fifty-four, Redondo Beach, California, marketing strategist: "Around 2000, my father was diagnosed with Alzheimer's disease. Unfortunately, his decline has accelerated in the last couple of years, and in 2008 he began being assisted through a hospice program.

"Doctors use a 0 to 30 scale to describe the level of cognition in patients. My dad was at a 20 or 21 level seven years ago. Now, at age eighty-eight, his level is around 10. He requires 24/7 care, including hand-feeding. He is pretty much immobile. He has to be lifted from the bed to the wheelchair. He's had no exercise in at least a year, and there are only very limited moments of awareness/consciousness. He has very, very limited moments of being in the present.

"The hospice doctors visit him monthly and monitor his health and overall condition. For the past several years, they have prescribed only two medications for him—one for the Alzheimer's and the other to regulate his blood pressure. He had been taking hypertension medication for years as well.

"At the end of 2008, I put a grounded sheet in my father's bed and he has slept grounded ever since. Six months or so later, the doctors observed that his blood pressure had returned to normal. They didn't understand how this could happen with someone who had no mobility. My father couldn't walk or talk. Consequently, they took him off his blood pressure medicine.

"Another unusual thing also occurred. He hasn't developed a single bedsore despite the fact he's sleeping perhaps 85 percent of the time. That's rather uncommon for someone so thoroughly bedridden. Bedsores develop when you don't move, and of course there's limited circulation. He didn't have bedsores before, but earlier on in the disease he was moving or being moved around. Since there is a radical decline in functionality toward the final stages of the disease, the doctors are surprised that there are no bedsores."

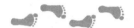

Jim Schmedding, sixty-three, Solana Beach, California, real estate broker: "I started sleeping grounded in the beginning of 2008, a time when I was coping with many health issues, high blood pressure being one of them. My pressure was up to 160/90, and there were times when the systolic pressure (top number) was hitting 185 and 190. The doctors had me on a bunch of medications to pull down the blood pressure to a level they could deal with.

"I was also taking Coumadin for an irregular heartbeat I had developed over the years. I could feel it racing at times and other times pausing for maybe five or more seconds. That obviously creates quite a lot of concern. You tend to get lightheaded or pass out when that happens. I've had moments where I had to pull off the road. To help prevent this situation, my doctors gave me a pacemaker.

"After the first month of grounding, my requirement for Coumadin changed significantly, to the point where the medication was cut in half. The doctors have kept me at that level as a stroke prevention strategy.

"Even with the pacemaker I would still have heart rhythm incidents about once a week. After I started Earthing, the incidents dropped off to maybe once a quarter. I think my whole cardiovascular system has been affected by it. I'm more relaxed. There's not as much tension in the system.

"My blood pressure also improved after grounding. It went down to about 140/80 or so. Then I went on a diet and started losing a lot of weight. Much of my problem with blood pressure is related to weight. I have always been big. I played professional football when I was younger. After my playing days, I added a lot of fat. I went from a playing weight of about 265 all the way up to 340 at the peak. Over the years I tried to lose weight many times but always had difficulty. I was dealing with stress in my life and the weight just kind of kept creeping up, no matter what I tried to do. My new diet emphasizes fruit and vegetables, with a little bit of protein, and that has helped me steadily get my weight down. It's now around 245. My blood pressure is 120/70. I've been able to reduce the blood pressure medication quite a bit. Ever since I became grounded, I'm much more relaxed and calmer than I have ever been. That's made a lot of difference, including I believe helping me to lose weight. My body reacts differently.

"I've had anemia over the years. My hemoglobin counts have always been kind of stressed. After grounding, the red blood cell count is still low, but the doctors are surprised at the size of them. My red blood cells are about twice the size of what normal guys have. The doctors found that quite unique and said it allows me to process oxygen better and deliver nutrients as if I had a higher hemoglobin count. The blood cells are seemingly functioning better.

"These doctors have been treating me for thirty years, and they were never really optimistic about my chances. Now I've become the new book for them. There's no protocol for me. They don't know how to explain any of this. The changes in my blood really threw them off. I told them the only thing that's changed in my life is sleeping grounded. I gave them some information on it. Their response was: 'Whatever you're doing, keep doing it, because it's working very well.'

"One other health issue I have been dealing with is lymphoma. I've had it for thirty years. Before I started grounding myself I underwent chemotherapy and then soon afterward I received a bone marrow transplant. I spent a lot of time recovering and sleeping on grounded sheets after the procedure. My blood tests looked very good. The doctors were really surprised that I responded as well as I did."

Note: Earthing has no effect on a pacemaker other than that which would occur naturally when standing barefoot on the Earth.

EARTHING—A NATURAL "BLOOD THINNER?"

In the fall of 2008, I invited a group of colleagues to my home in Connecticut to participate in an unusual experiment. There were twelve of us.

We were clinical physicians, Ph.D.s working in the medical field, nurses, an attorney, two artists, a personal trainer, and Clint Ober.

The experiment involved taking a drop of blood before and after forty minutes of grounding via electrode patches, and then examining the fresh, unstained blood under a darkfield microscope. These microscopes, used by many doctors, particularly in the field of alternative medicine, divert light through the optical system so that details appear light against a dark background. This technique allows viewing of "live time" cellular dynamics and conditions of blood not normally analyzed through routine tests.

The pictures shocked me and all my guests. The after-grounding pictures showed that people's blood dramatically changes within a short period of time after an individual is in contact with the Earth. Specifically, there were considerably fewer formations of red blood cells associated with clumping and clotting. The blood appeared to be thinner.

In my informal home experiment, all of us present except one person in the room had various degrees of red "ketchupy" blood before Earthing. The sole exception, the one with the best blood of anyone present, before or after grounding, was Clint Ober—someone who has been consistently Earthing himself day and night for years!

To all of us, the results suggested that individuals with heart disease and inflammatory thick blood (typical in cardiovascular disease and diabetes) may reap huge health benefits from simply Earthing themselves on a regular basis. From a cardiology standpoint, if you can thin the typical ketchup-like blood of heart patients and people with diabetes in the direction of the consistency of wine, as our simple experiment showed, you remove a colossal risk factor for heart attack and stroke.

"Blood is thicker than water" is an old saying, expressing the importance of family ties. But in the medical world, you don't want thick blood. Earthing may be a natural way to keep it nice and thin. Cardiologists use the term viscosity to describe blood thickness. Blood viscosity, an overlooked element in blood tests, has become an emerging major marker for identifying the risk of arterial disease. The thicker your blood, the slower it flows through your circulatory system to bring oxygen and vital nutrients to the cells of your body, and the greater the risk of forming clots. Coumadin is a widely used medication for thinning the blood and helping prevent clotting.

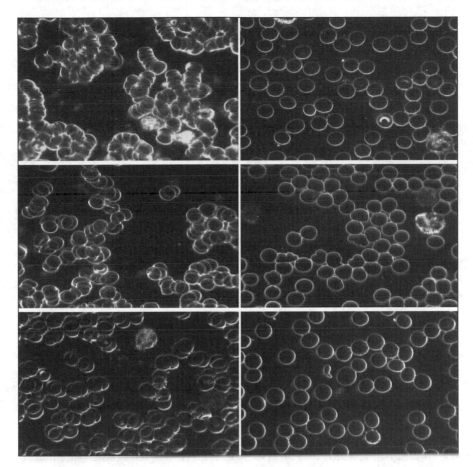

Figure 11-1. The reproductions above represent darkfield microscope images of blood taken from three individuals in attendance at Dr. Sinatra's house just before and after forty minutes of grounding. The before images are on the left, the after on the right. The pictures clearly show a dramatic thinning and decoupling of blood cells.

Note: Because of Earthing's effect on blood viscosity, individuals taking Coumadin should first talk to their doctor before grounding. Although we have no evidence for it, it is possible that the combination of Earthing and Coumadin could excessively thin the blood. For this reason, heart patients taking Coumadin should ground themselves only with the knowledge and approval of their physicians. With such approval, grounding should start minimally, with perhaps a barefoot walk in the park or for an hour or two while watching TV in the house while in contact with some kind of an indoor Earthing device. Patients' blood should be monitored more frequently than normal to determine whether at some point, because of the Earthing, the medication dosage can be safely reduced. Earthing sessions can be increased slowly, and if safe, individuals should consider sleeping grounded. I urge any patient taking Coumadin to exercise caution in this manner.

More Fascinating Evidence

The informal experiment in my home inspired a study in 2009 to investigate further whether Earthing can indeed influence red blood cell clumping as we saw in the darkfield images. I was particularly intrigued to find out if the results were reproducible. With this goal in mind, I set up a study with Gaetan Chevalier, Ph.D., the California electrophysiologist who has been involved in other Earthing research. We designed an experiment to measure not only blood clumping but also something called the zeta potential. You've likely never heard of zeta potential. Most people haven't. It relates to the degree of negative charge on the surface of a red blood cell.

We selected ten healthy individuals—none of whom took any medication—to participate in the study. They came individually to a health clinic in Southern California and sat comfortably in a reclining chair while they were grounded for two hours. Grounded electrode patches were placed on their feet and hands, just as had been done in previous studies. Blood samples were taken before and after two hours of continual grounding.

When the blood was analyzed, we were quite surprised. We had been expecting a small improvement in the zeta potential, perhaps by 30 percent. Instead, we found an improvement of 270 percent on average!

Just what does this mean to you? The results strongly suggest the discovery of a natural solution for blood thinning, an option of great interest not just for cardiologists like me, but also for any physician concerned about the relationship of blood viscosity and inflammation.

According to the scientific literature on the subject, the healthy range for the zeta potential is between -9.3 millivolts (mV) and -15 mV, with an average of -12.5 mV. In our experiment, two hours of grounding improved the average zeta potential of the ten participates from a rather depressed level of −5.28 mV before Earthing to a healthy −14.26 mV. My understanding is that blood *low* in zeta potential is more apt to be sludgy and thick, flow less freely, and have a greater risk of clumping and clotting. By comparison, a higher zeta potential translates to a higher negative charge of the particles in the blood, such as the red blood cells. That means they repel each other more readily, creating more elbow room between them, and better flow. Blood vessels are like highways. You want the traffic moving smoothly and fluidly. You don't want traffic jams.

Numbers aside, the impression we have is that Earthing apparently alters and normalizes blood voltage rapidly, improving the zeta potential and viscosity. Technically, we exposed small amounts of blood to an electric field and observed, with the use of a darkfield microscope, how much red blood cells moved in a certain period of time. We did this before and after two hours of grounding. The red blood cells barely moved in our observations of blood taken before grounding. After grounding, they moved in a rapid manner. In addition, there were considerably more clumps of red cells in the before pictures than in the after pictures.

Taken together, these results suggest better circulation, blood flow, and viscosity—thinner, more mobile blood. That's what any cardiologist likes to see.

Research on zeta potential is limited, but it seems to me that this concept has the potential to serve as a new gold standard for determining inflammation in the blood, and by extension, provide a superb and accurate yardstick for measuring the overall health of an individual. This concept was unknown to me until only recently. Cardiologists are by and large unfamiliar with the bioelectrical nature of blood. So due scientific diligence must be done in the form of careful study. We can't say much more at this point, but the implications are extremely promising and certainly warrant more research. We are planning a bigger study to confirm our preliminary findings.

As Dr. Chevalier told me, if Earthing affects blood as we have seen in this pilot investigation, that means Earthing really affects the metabolism of the entire body at the cellular level. This further supports our hypothesis that grounded people have a different physiology than people who are ungrounded. As more research rolls out, we may find that we need to rewrite physiology books!

MY BOTTOM LINE

During more than several decades in medical practice, I have witnessed firsthand how broadening my treatment options into an integrated approach—using effective combinations of conventional and alternative medicine—has dramatically improved the health of patients. Pharmaceuticals and surgery are so often lifesaving in acute situations. So, too, the use of key nutritional supplements and mind/body techniques can powerfully influence both failing hearts and failing cardiac function. For me, it's a no-brainer to use the best of both worlds. For more than twenty years, I have been routinely prescribing supplements—such as CoQ10. Most of that time, my colleagues in cardiology chided me for doing so. It wasn't the accepted way cardiology was practiced, they implied. I told them that many of my patients were still alive and thriving because I did.

I feel the same way now about grounding, a simple and safe remedy that seemingly and surprisingly addresses so much of what ails us. It is perhaps the most natural prescription we can recommend to any patient—a perfectly natural adjunct to any clinical strategy. I am totally comfortable telling someone to go barefoot and/or sleep grounded. I do it myself. It's almost amusing to think that in our pursuit of expensive high-tech solutions, we all have access to a low-tech solution right there on the ground we walk on. Just connect to it one way or another, and heal yourself.

Electromedicine and the use of healing energies have interested me for many years. I feel this is the future of medicine. How appropriate that our very own planet may give us—the planet dwellers—the most basic healing vibe of all. What a gift!

CHAPTER 12

The Feminine Connection: Earthing and Women

Women seem to get it.

They seem to respond intuitively and immediately to the "barefoot connection" and to the healing and energy of Mother Earth. This is not in any way a criticism of the masculine mind, but simply an observation based on years of demonstrating and explaining the concept of Earthing to thousands of people.

"Connect to the Earth and heal" was the way one group of women, in chorus, described Earthing some years ago.

Women seem to enjoy kicking off their shoes at the desk or at home, something you will rarely see a man do. It's not so much that the shoes are uncomfortable, but rather more of a primordial and harmonious connection to the Earth that women may feel more intimately than men.

Women are caregivers by nature. Clint Ober has found that after experiencing the benefits of Earthing, women want to go out and tell everyone in their circle of family and friends. By comparison, men generally want to know how it works.

There is also an appearance factor here. One woman with multiple sclerosis who participated in a one-day Earthing study visited the restroom at the end of the day and then rushed back to the testing center all excited. "I look different," she said. "Like I used to look years ago." Other women have made this comment, even after just a half hour of grounding. And after sleeping grounded for a period of time, women often say they feel better and look better. They say their skin has more radiance, their eyes are brighter, and they have more vitality. The impact on feeling and appearance is likely from a combination of things: elimination of an electron deficiency, better sleep, reduced stress and pain, and more natural and balanced functioning within the body. The feedback suggests that these factors work to help normalize many ongoing health issues and may even be helpful in the struggle against weight gain.

Earthing may contribute on the weight front in part by making you feel more relaxed and normalizing your level of cortisol (the stress hormone). People under stress often have a hard time following a healthy diet. They will frequently eat the wrong things to fill an emotional need or because of lack of time to prepare something healthy for themselves.

The body produces excess cortisol in times of physical and psychological stress. The hormone revs up fat and carbohydrate metabolism for fast energy. Too much stress and too much cortisol in the system can boost the appetite and, according to some studies, promote weight gain. What's more, stress and cortisol can promote fat deposition around the middle, a highly unhealthy and unsightly buildup referred to as abdominal adiposity. The problem with this form of belly fat is that it produces inflammatory chemicals and is a paramount feature of the metabolic syndrome that leads to cardiovascular disease and diabetes. We haven't specifically researched Earthing's effect on weight yet, but quite a few people have remarked about finding it easier to lose weight and keep weight off.

Hormones are a central—and often confusing—concern to women throughout much of their lives. No research has been done to date regarding hormones and Earthing other than a pivotal study on cortisol that we described earlier in Chapter 4. It is well known that hormones work in harmony with each other, even though we are far from understanding all the complex give-and-take and up-and-down interactions. Often, when the body's production of one hormone is off, others are affected, kind of like a domino effect. Cortisol is a close steroid relative of progesterone and more distantly to estrogen. So there could be some impact here that has not been measured yet. Something positive is happening, though. We have received feedback from many women describing relief from debilitating symptoms of PMS and menopause, sometimes quite rapidly.

IN THEIR OWN WORDS

In the original cortisol study published in 2004, the participants provided comments on their health issues prior to and after eight weeks of sleeping grounding. Following is a summary of feedback from five of the female participants. Their responses represent a vision of possibilities from Earthing after just a short period of time. Keep in mind that each person is an individual and is likely to respond differently from the next person. However, the feedback is fairly typical of many other observations made over the years.

Participant No. 1, fifty-three years old, menopausal

Pre-Study Complaints

- Difficulty going to sleep.
- Wakes up two to three times a night for last three years.
- Muscle cramps in legs.
- Chronic muscle pain throughout body.
- Hot flashes.

End of Study Feedback

- "Fall asleep faster and easier."
- "Neck pain lessened."
- "Leg and foot cramps have lessened."
- "Arm and lower back pain gone by the very first week."
- "TMJ (temporomandibular joint disorder) problem significantly improved."
- "Reduction in hot flashes."

Participant No. 2, twenty-four years old

Pre-Study Complaints

- Trouble sleeping for seventeen years; takes a long time to fall asleep; wakes up after several hours and can't sleep again; wakes up exhausted.

- Daily headaches.

- Migraines one week before period.

- Menstrual cramps, mood swings, bloating, irritability, depression, and weight gain.

- Digestion: bloating, nausea, diarrhea, gas, and constipation.

End of Study Feedback

- "By the third night, decreased time to go to sleep and slept through the night."

- "Able to fall back asleep within a few minutes after waking up, and no more nightmares."

- "Wake up refreshed instead of exhausted."

- "No more daily headaches."

- "Decreased PMS, including food cravings, bloating, and depression."

- "Digestion improved with less bloating, constipation, and nausea."

Participant No. 3, fifty-two years old, menopausal

Pre-Study Complaints

- Sleeps very lightly.

- Wakes up feeling tense several times during the night.

- Wakes up feeling tired in morning; feel tired all day.

- Pain in left hip, sporadic for several years.

- Allergies (food and airborne) since age thirteen.

- Digestion: gas.

End of Study Feedback

- "Have felt more rested and feel like I need an hour less sleep per night."

- "Deeper relaxation."

- "Stopped having any pain at all in my left hip."

- "First few days, I experienced tingling and heat in areas of my previous physical injuries—similar to an acupuncture treatment. After about three days, these vague feelings subsided."

- "Allergies have definitely lessened."
- "Better digestion."
- "I noticed that I stopped clenching my jaw at night."
- The participant reported that her husband, who was not part of the study, but who was sleeping grounded next to her, "began sleeping fewer hours, has more energy, and has stopped snoring."

Participant No. 4, forty-two years old

Pre-Study Complaints

- Trouble falling asleep; light restless sleep.
- Wakes up feeling tired; also, trouble waking up from naps.
- Fibromyalgia since 1992 car accident; a lot of joint pain in arms, legs, ankles.
- Gastrointestinal upset; gas.

End of Study Feedback

- "The general quality of my sleep improved; not immediate, but a gradual change."
- "Sleeping much deeper."
- "A lot less fatigue because of less pain."
- "My fibromyalgia has improved considerably because of diminished pain and fatigue; the joint pain is gone, with occasional pain in the left arm."
- "I am feeling much better, I haven't been sick at all."

Participant No. 5, forty-four years old

Pre-Study Complaints

- Trouble sleeping; wakes up two to three times each night with physical discomfort.

- Numb fingers on left hand for last four months; carpal tunnel syndrome.

- Bad cramps, breast tenderness, mood swings, weight gain, painful heavy periods, and uterine fibroids for many years.

- Hot flashes at night (or maybe night sweats).

- History of anxiety attacks.

End of Study Feedback

- "Gradually sleeping better"

- "Two episodes of waking up between 4:30 and 5:30 a.m. with anxiety that subsides by early afternoon.

- "Less numbness in hand and fingers, especially at night; not needing to wear a brace at night."

- "Menstrual periods not as severe; cramps not as strong."

- "Feeling better physically and emotionally."

TWO STORIES OF RELIEF FROM MENSTRUAL AND MENOPAUSAL MISERY

Amanda Ward, N.D., thirty, Encinitas, California, naturopathic doctor: "I started Earthing myself and had phenomenal results. My sleep was deeper. When I would become run down, I would wrap myself up in a grounding sheet and recover quickly. However, the most dramatic effect was on my own menstrual issues. I used to have horrific PMS with heavy periods and severe cramping and pain. Nothing I tried was helping me much, even though I have a lot of tools at my disposal as a health practitioner. At times the situation would be debilitating enough so that I had to stay at home.

"After about two months of Earthing, I started to notice an improvement. Then every month my periods would become a little better. In about a year, my menstrual difficulties completely resolved. Now, I might get a bit of irritability, but all the physical symptoms are gone.

"As I began to see the improvements in my own life, I began recommending Earthing to patients. I do a lot of hormone balancing and nutrition to support women's health issues. I use a broad array of methods, so it is hard to say exactly which treatment is helping the most. However, patients have told me that they feel more balanced with Earthing than they do on the other programs alone. My clinical impression is that women who do the Earthing along with bioidentical hormones definitely seem to have a superior experience. There is a lot of synergy here. Hormonal imbalances are so prevalent, and Earthing seems to be such a simple and profound tool to smooth out those imbalances.

"I have seen particularly good results with perimenopause and menopause, with reduction of symptoms like hot flashes, night sweats, insomnia, and irritability.

"Some of the mothers in my practice have told me that they have used Earthing sheets and helped their kids recover faster from cold and flu symptoms. I've heard this feedback even from women whose children have weaker immune systems and tend to be sick frequently. The mothers will take the grounding sheet they themselves use and wrap up the kids in it when they are watching TV. If the kids sleep grounded, I've heard, they sleep a lot better."

Dale Teplitz, M.A., fifty-five, San Diego, California, health researcher: "Ever since my periods began at age thirteen, and until I was forty-five, I suffered routinely with severe PMS and menstrual symptoms. In the week prior to each period, I experienced gradually increasing water retention, food cravings, headaches, and weight gain. I was irritable. My skin was itchy and uncomfortable. My body ached and felt painful to the touch. For several nights prior to every period, I could not sleep. Over the years, I took diuretics to help with the water retention and sleeping pills for those difficult nights.

"PMS also affected my personality and relationships; I had emotional ups and downs, anxiety, and often felt depressed. Medication left me feeling emotionally numb.

"Once my period began, the PMS symptoms would go away to be replaced by severe cramps and heavy bleeding. The pain and fatigue often prevented me from working. I lived on anti-inflammatories during this time, which disturbed my digestion.

"At the age of forty-five, I started sleeping grounded. One month later, all the PMS symptoms went away: the cramps, fatigue, bloating, irritability, cravings, sleeplessness, headaches, weight gain, and depression. I was astounded. After thirty-two years, they stopped suddenly. In one stroke, I was able to eliminate the sleeping pills, diuretics, antiinflammatories, and other medications. I was free of symptoms, and I felt like a new person.

"Two years later, I entered menopause, at around the same age my mother had. I was feeling a bit anxious about what might lie ahead because I had heard horror stories from other women. It seemed that those who had a lot of PMS issues had the most difficulty going through menopause.

"To my surprise, I sailed into menopause effortlessly. I had a gradual decrease in the frequency and duration of periods until they eventually disappeared. I did not experience sleeplessness or hot flashes (other than mild and brief hot flashes, which I determined were related to certain foods or red wine) or any of the other hormonal-type mood swings all my friends reported. Some of my friends have had menopause symptoms for more than ten years now, well into their sixties.

"Another thing that amazes me is that when I was in my early forties, I had been diagnosed with osteopenia, a condition in which bone density is below normal and may lead to osteoporosis. For several years in a row, I had a dual energy x-ray absorptionmetry scan, or DEXA scan, that showed decreased density of my thigh and ankle bones. When I was tested again at age forty-eight, after sleeping grounded for three years, the osteopenia was gone. I was tested again at fifty-two, and it was still gone! My bone density looked great.

"I am convinced that Earthing took away my symptoms of PMS, cramps, and menopause. I doubt that indigenous women who live directly on the Earth are troubled with symptoms of hormone imbalance. I can't imagine how much better my life would have been if I had learned about Earthing thirty years sooner, but nobody knew about it then. So I consider myself lucky to have heard about it at all. I could have continued suffering much longer."

"I HAVE MY HEALTH BACK"

Elizabeth Hughes, Ph.D., fifty-three, Palm Springs, California, former corporate executive: "At age twenty-one, I developed fever, sore throat, muscle soreness, headaches, swollen glands, and fatigue. My doctor thought I had a case of mononucleosis, a viral condition that frequently strikes young adults. I spent a lot of time in bed and out of commission for the next twenty-five or so years, with one variation or another of some sickness. It seemed to me that my doctors used different names for the shifting symptoms according to whatever mystery disease was in vogue at the time: things like chronic fatigue, Epstein-Barr virus, fibromyalgia, and Ramsay Hunt syndrome. One doctor thought I had MS. I didn't.

"I was stuck in a system where doctors have great intentions but few explanations about how you got sick and very little to heal you with. A few doctors said it was all in my head and offered antidepressants and psychotherapy. Early on a team of six interns reviewed my case and said they didn't know what was wrong even though my symptoms were obvious.

"Many chemicals made me sick. For a long time, I couldn't set foot in a hairdresser's salon or department store. New synthetic fabrics, carpets, outgassing solvents, and volatile compounds were a problem.

"I did all I could to get well. When conventional treatments failed, I tried the alternatives. I drank 16 ounces of wheat grass juice daily to detoxify myself. I ate pure organic uncooked food. I had my amalgam fillings removed to get rid of mercury in my body. I got some temporary relief from all these things, but nothing lasting or really substantial.

"Despite ongoing health issues, I managed to earn a Ph.D. in psychology and work in corporate America at a very high level. When I got very sick, I just had to go on disability and drop out for a while.

"I was always searching for an answer, but I could not find it. I even joined support groups with other women who had the same kind of complaints. It was so bad and so hopeless for some of those women that they committed suicide.

"If I had the money back that I spent on all this, on doctors and healers, I would be rich. After some temporary relief from one thing or another, I would go back to work so I could earn enough money to pay for treating the next episode.

"In 2005, I went to the emergency room with sharp pain in my ear. The doctor thought I might be developing Ramsay Hunt syndrome, a condition that produces severe pain, facial paralysis, herpetic blisters, loss of taste, and vertigo. The cause is thought to be the same virus behind shingles. They shot me up with something for the pain and gave me antidepressants. The relief was temporary.

"Shortly after that episode, I met Clint Ober and got grounded. Within six weeks I was a new person. I was amazed. Shocked is actually a better word. There was no more pain in my body. My symptoms of mononucleosis, chronic fatigue, fibromyalgia, or whatever was plaguing me were gone. I also didn't suffer anymore with tender, painful breasts, something always present during menstruation. The hot flashes I was beginning to experience with increasing frequency as I entered menopause subsided and then disappeared. I have my health back and without any medication."

REGULARITY RETURNS TO RUNNER

Amenorrhea and irregular periods are fairly common among high-intensity runners and dancers, activities that emphasize leanness. The experience below of one runner, a former state high-school champion, raises the possibility that Earthing may improve menstrual irregularities among physically active girls and women.

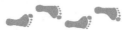

Brianna Anderson-Gregg, twenty-three, Springfield, Oregon, long-distance runner: "My periods used to be very irregular. I would frequently miss a month.

"After I started sleeping grounded, my periods normalized and I don't think I have missed a month since. That's probably about two years now. I never really thought about it, but then I realized at one point I had become regular.

"All the girls I have run and trained with for a long time have had at least a situation where they miss once in a while. One of them didn't have her period until she was out of high school and took a break from running."

RETURN TO DANCING AFTER CHILDBIRTH, KNEE PAIN

Olivia Biera, thirty, Los Angeles, California, healing arts business consultant: "I've been involved for years professionally as a traditional Aztec dancer, performing at festivals and historical locations. This is very vigorous dancing, very lower-body intensive. After having my daughter in 2005, I was anxious to get back into it, but I didn't have the same flexibility and muscularity that I had had before. I think I pushed myself too hard trying to come back and did something to my right knee that caused chronic inflammation. An MRI showed no tear, just deep inflammation. The knee was like one big swollen balloon that hurt badly. It was difficult to walk up stairs. Driving and carrying my baby made it worse. In addition, my right hip was also giving me a lot of trouble after childbirth.

"I had to do something. Massage and other therapies I tried weren't working. It was almost impossible to stretch. At one point in 2007, I was two weeks away from explorative knee surgery. That's when I started sleeping and working grounded. I immediately noticed an ability to sleep through the pain. From one week to the next, the inflammation began to go down. After about six weeks, it was 30 to 40 percent less—and that was without icing. I was so busy in my work that when I would get home to my little girl, I just didn't have time or energy to ice the knee as I should. I no longer needed to sleep with a pillow between my legs to ease the pain. The pain was just slowly slipping away. I never had that surgery.

"After about a year, the knee and hip were about 90 percent normal, and I was able to start dancing again. And a few more months later, everything was 100 percent.

"Perhaps the biggest surprise is what happened to my nicotine craving. No matter how many good health practices I followed, like yoga and good diet, I couldn't kick the craving. I'd been smoking for thirteen years when I became pregnant. I quit. It's not that I smoked a lot, but at the end of my workday I had a craving for cigarettes that would drive me nuts. I would smoke one cigarette and then maybe another cigarette. After six weeks, the craving was gone, and I haven't smoked since.

"I also experienced a definite release of emotional stresses. At the time I started grounding, I had a lot going on in my life. I definitely noticed right off the bat a sense of rejuvenation and emotional 'grounding.' I was grounded physically and that grounded me emotionally and even spiritually, in the sense of being connected to the Earth.

"My sleep pattern changed as well. I recognized quickly that I was sleeping deeper. I also noticed something with my daughter that was quite interesting. She always used to fall asleep in a curled, fetal position. She would typically roll around the bed until she found the perfect curved position to sleep in. Then, at age two, when she started to sleep grounded, she fell asleep straight as a board—the very first night. It was like a magnet pulled her into the sheets, and she slept totally relaxed. She also functions at a level way above her age group, and I believe strongly that has a lot to do with sleeping grounded. She is four now with great concentration and does things that second graders do.

"At my office, we use grounded floor pads. There are computers, printers, telephones, and electronic equipment, which probably emit a lot of electromagnetic pollution. I myself used to get tired. Not after I began working grounded. I grounded the whole office and there has been a tremendous increase in productivity and in terms of being alert, not having computer drain, staying with the game, and getting it done."

A PREGNANCY STORY

Stephanie Okeafor, thirty-three, Paradise Valley, Arizona, personal trainer and microcurrent therapist: "My husband and I have been sleeping grounded for more than five years, and sleeping better as a result. The most dramatic thing for me has been the effect on my pregnancy, and particularly the first trimester. This was my first pregnancy.

"I am a very active person and follow a rigorous fitness routine. When I became pregnant, I didn't run as much, but I was still doing the same intensity of lifting, lunges, and cross-training activities. I realized quickly that I was okay in the moment doing these workouts, but afterward— within the next hour or so—I would feel pretty exhausted.

"I would go home and say okay, I'm pregnant, I'll take a nap. I need to take care of myself. But I never really needed a big nap. I would lie down on the grounding sheet, and after twenty minutes I would get up, feeling completely alert and rested, and ready to go.

Is There an Earthing-Pregnancy Connection?

Russell Whitten, D.C., forty, Santa Barbara, California, chiropractor:
"I started grounding patients back in 2000, and I had some great feedback from many of them. A few told me, however, they didn't know if it was working or not. I began to realize they no longer had pain and had forgotten they had it before, unless I mentioned it.

"My patients have frequently told me that their dreams become more vivid when they start to sleep grounded and, in some cases, almost psychedelic-like.

"Perhaps the most amazing Earthing story I have witnessed involves my own wife, Joey. She had not been able to get pregnant during the eight years of her first marriage. Then, for the first six years of our relationship, she was still unable to conceive. From a medical standpoint, everything appeared normal, but it just never happened. In 2000, we started sleeping grounded, and within a month she became pregnant, for the first time, at the age of thirty-five.

"In my opinion, there was nothing else but grounding that could explain it. I had been giving her chiropractic adjustments for a couple of years at that point so that wasn't what made the difference.

"Within six months of meeting Clint Ober, I had grounded roughly fifty of my patients' beds. It was soon reported back to me that several of my patients who were in their forties had become pregnant after starting to sleep grounded. Each had had their children in their twenties and now years later were able to conceive again. It seemed like more than just a coincidence to me. I also heard that women's periods became less symptomatic and their hormonal systems seemed to normalize. There may be great potential here for the fertility industry.

"Joey gave birth in April 2001 to a boy. He was born at home on our grounded bed. We named him Tiger because my wife had had a vivid dream while pregnant that she had a tiger in her belly. We wanted to create a name that said something about him and his spirit.

"Tiger has slept grounded from the start and has had excellent health. As a toddler he was considerably taller than most kids his age, while both my wife and I are of average size. He was speaking much earlier than expected. By eighteen months, he had a vocabulary of a couple of hundred words and was making short sentences. It could be that the Earthing had something to do with all that as well."

"I have had a very easy pregnancy compared to most women I've talked to. It's my first so I don't have anything for personal comparison. I haven't had any sickness at all. I've worked out the entire time. I've had excellent energy except for after the workouts. My friends comment about my energy and activity level. Also, it's been over 100 degrees every day for the last half of my pregnancy. People wonder how I'm doing so well with all the heat.

"I'm absolutely sure that being fit helps the situation. Conceiving when you're in good shape puts you ahead in the game compared to someone who starts out her pregnancy not in shape. However, I have a lot of friends who are in great shape, and they've had a hard time throughout their pregnancy. I know each pregnancy is different, but getting great sleep and grounding for an extra twenty minutes here and there during the day I'm sure is a big reason for my energy level."

Note: Stephanie had a home birth in October 2009. The rest of her story was filled in by her husband Chike, a professional football player: "It all went beautifully. Stephanie rocketed through it. She was very powerful. I was awestruck. Our midwife was very impressed. I was able to catch my daughter and cut the umbilical cord. She came out and her eyes were clear and alert. She started feeding pretty much right away. Stephanie is six foot and I am six foot five, and Anaya Louise, our daughter, weighed in at 10 pounds, 4 ounces. Mother and baby are doing very well. Both are staying grounded."

CHAPTER 13

The Sports Connection: Earthing in Action

Biophysicist James Oschman tells the story of a friend who ran in a marathon. Part of the way through the race, he developed a very painful blister on his foot. Recalling the great barefoot runners from Africa, who have dominated the marathon-racing scene for years, he yanked off his shoes and pushed on without them. Not only was he able to finish the race without pain, he was also very surprised at the end to find that his blister was completely gone.

If that seems hard to believe, consider the most dramatic application of Earthing: the experience of recent victorious U.S.-sponsored teams in cycling's premier event, the Tour de France. The success of grounding in one of the most challenging racing competitions in the world is extraordinary.

The grounding-cycling story starts in 2003, when Jeff Spencer, D.C., a prominent sports medicine specialist based in Pasadena, California, contacted Clint Ober. He had heard about Earthing from a San Diego doctor and was intrigued by the concept. Dr. Spencer, a former Olympic cyclist, works with elite athletes functioning at the highest level of performance and applies cutting-edge methods to support optimum health and enhance recovery from exertion and injury. This was his assignment during five Tour de France competitions. During four of them, 2003 to 2005, and again in 2007, he utilized Earthing.

EARTHING AT THE TOUR DE FRANCE

"I've had the good fortune of working with many athletes at the highest level in terms of getting them to the top of their game and keeping them there. You can't imagine what a challenge that is when the sports event is the Tour de France. My No. 1 job was to make sure that the riders showed up everyday, at the starting line, 100 percent mentally and physically ready for the rides of their lives. On the other side of that was to make sure that we had very aggressive recovery strategies so that they could survive this inhumane event called the Tour de France. In doing so, I had to develop as compressed a timeline for injury and full-body recovery as possible. The challenge gave me tremendous flexibility in putting together a 'tool kit' that would give us a competitive advantage. In the Tours that I worked, we lost only four riders—one to a broken arm, one to severe tendonitis, another to a broken arm, and the other to a broken hand. Otherwise, all the other riders finished, which is really unheard of in this sport.

"Le Tour Terrible"

The Tour de France is among the most brutal athletic events in the world—comparable to running three marathons a day for twenty-one straight days. Racers may climb as much as a total of 30,000 feet in a single day's stage. That's six miles straight up. The race covers 2,100 miles on the ground and ranges from sea level to 8,700 feet.

In July, when the race is run, the weather is very hot in France. The narrow asphalt roads over which the Tour is run start to crack, blister, and soften, making the going extremely treacherous. Falling on that kind of surface is like landing on a cheese grater. Cyclists suffer massive abrasions affectionately known as "road rash."

The traffic around the racers as they go from stage to stage is intense. There are more than 170 cyclists racing in a very crowded pack. They are shadowed by a chaotic convoy of support vehicles carrying mechanics, spare bicycles and parts, as well as vehicles with Tour officials, media, and security personnel. The combination of cyclists, high speeds, narrow roads, cars, and motorcycles is a recipe for mishaps. Crashes are common and can cause serious physical trauma.

"As a doctor who has worked with some of the best of the best in the sports world, I've found that it's essential to never allow yourself to believe that what you did before is any guarantee of future success. So, by definition, I'm always looking for new innovations that will take me to the next level and give me that competitive edge over the competition. I am continually remodeling my ultimate clinical 'tool box' so as to stay current with state-of-the-art equipment and methods.

"When I first heard about Earthing, it sounded very interesting to me. I had never heard of it before, but it sounded like something that might be useful for what I do. I contacted the developer of the technology (Clint Ober) and asked to meet with him. When we talked, it became clear to me that if Earthing did what he said it was supposed to do, it could give the Tour cyclists a tremendous advantage.

"Earthing wouldn't change anything I normally did. And all somebody had to do is lay down and go to sleep or relax like they would normally do. This would help them sleep and relax, so I was told. This was very appealing. I knew that when I would spend time outdoors with my feet in the sand or I'd walk at the beach with my feet close to the water, I would feel a lot better.

"But I first had to try the technology on myself. I was not willing to use anything for my patients that I didn't know worked from my own firsthand experience. For about five years, I had been suffering with the consequences of mercury poisoning. At one point, my health was quite debilitated. I had been receiving treatment for it and was improving gradually. I was getting better. But after grounding myself one night, I felt a significant improvement. When I awoke the next morning, I felt much better. I had more energy. I had had difficulty concentrating before, but now I had greater clarity of thinking. I had less pain. Less irritability. My body felt like it had been washed from inside out. After three or four nights of sleeping better and feeling better, I knew that this was something for real. I recognized that this is something that could have tremendous value not just for me, but also for my patients and the cyclists at the Tour de France.

"I was, to say the least, impressed. I asked Clint if he could create a prototype system for me to take and use at the Tour de France. The challenge is that the Tour is so difficult mentally and physically that the riders have a hard time sleeping. And if you don't sleep, you don't recover. If you don't recover, the body breaks down, the mind goes down, and you can unnecessarily get injured or sick, which is catastrophic for a top Tour effort."

A Huge Difference

"Clint agreed and came up with a prototype system. It had a metallic snap at one end that connected to a wire that ran to an outside ground rod. Clint handmade all the wiring and taught me how to use the system. It was ready just in time for the 2003 Tour de France. And it made a huge difference. The severe mental and physical strain from daily competition needs to be discharged from the body while the rider is relaxing and recovering, so we need technology available at night in order that the rider gets up the next morning fully recovered.

"I saw the same experiences among the riders that I had experienced myself. They slept much better. And that's a big deal in a competition like this where cyclists have a very hard time sleeping because they are so overstimulated from the Tour's intensity and, ironically, often overtired. When they can't rest and sleep enough, they can break down. When trying to sustain high performance at this level, team physicians always wonder how they can improve sleep and take advantage of the sleep downtime. So Earthing was like an answer to my prayers. The riders reported less mental tension and stress. They felt calmer. Their decision-making was good. Their vitality and morale were really high."

Accelerated Healing

"We also applied Earthing, along with other treatments, to accelerate tissue repair and wound healing from injuries sustained during the competition. The results were phenomenal. The cyclists recovered much faster.

"The most dramatic case involved a cyclist in the 2005 Tour who suffered severe lacerations to his upper right arm after crashing through the rear window of a support car that had stopped abruptly (see Figure 13-1). He managed to make it to the finish line. He immediately received aggressive medical treatment and was taken to a local hospital for stitches. When I saw him on the team bus right after that day's Tour stage, he had shock written all over his face. His jersey and riding shorts were bloody. His arm had been tightly bandaged to stop the bleeding. When the bandages were removed, you could actually see the tendons and bones through the torn flesh. It looked like somebody had chopped up his arm with a carving

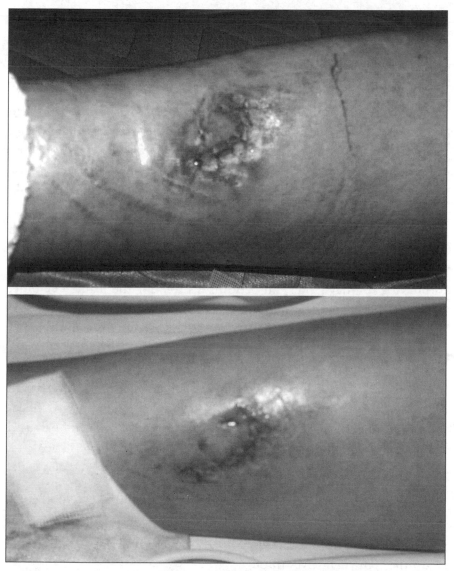

Figure 13-1. Rapid wound healing. Overnight grounding accelerated the healing of this, and many other similar cycling wounds. (*Photos courtesy of Jeff Spencer, D.C.*)

knife. Later at the hotel, we saw extensive stitches in his upper arm, as well as his elbow, hand, and chin. He had a large purple bruise on his leg, as if someone had hit him with a lead pipe. The team had serious reservations about whether he could continue in the Tour because of the extent of his injuries. Everybody doubted he would be able return to competition the next day.

"I asked for twelve hours—basically overnight—to try to help him heal enough to continue racing. I knew that Earthing could make a big difference. Everybody agreed it was worth a shot as long as he wasn't in danger of hurting himself further. So I applied multiple grounded electrodes to his arm and leg and he slept grounded that night, as he had throughout the competition. When he awoke the next day, there wasn't nearly the pain, redness, soreness, or swelling he had the night before. He didn't seem nearly as bad off as would be normally expected. He felt up to going out that day and racing. Our high hopes were that he could continue, finish the day's ride, and get stronger and heal more each subsequent day. I took the patches off him and gave him additional care with other techniques. I taped up his bruised leg, and he was rebandaged, and off he went to race that day's stage. It turned out that he was indeed able to put in a full day's ride and perform his role for the team. The other cyclists were overjoyed. He ultimately finished the competition and contributed to the team victory. To an outsider, his recovery was nothing less than miraculous.

"In my experience with Earthing, this kind of response is not surprising anymore. In many instances, I have seen an absence of what we regard as a normal inflammatory response. When individuals are grounded, injuries lack much—and I mean much—of the typical degree of pain and redness. Tissue repair is accelerated.

"At the end of the 2005 Tour, the team director asked me about the condition of the riders.

" 'They're doing great,' I said.

" 'What about tendonitis?' he asked. Cyclists have a high incidence of tendon inflammation in their legs because of the prolonged and intense strain they put themselves through.

" 'It wasn't a problem,' I said.

" 'Anybody sick?' he asked.

" 'No, everybody's good,' I answered.

"He shrugged and said, 'incredible.'

"Acute traumatic injury is common in the world of athletics, so Earthing is a great boon. Grounding helps minimize injury downtime and speed recovery. I know how long it takes to recover normally. And I also know what happens when an athlete is grounded. The changes in terms of body recovery from day to day, the ability to repair tissue, to recover from activity and the stresses and strains of the day, are amazing. To me, it's obvious that any athlete should make Earthing part of his or her regular wellness program.

"Earthing also appears to accelerate recovery from surgery, which, as far as the body is concerned, is basically a form of traumatic injury. One of my patients is a champion in Supercross, a wild and wooly sport where off-road motorcycles race in stadium dirt tracks filled with steep jumps and obstacles. My patient suffered a bad shoulder injury that required surgery. He was treated in a variety of ways to speed the healing process, including sleeping grounded. In three weeks, he was able to compete in a national event and win the competition. He made an amazingly rapid recovery."

Less Pain

"Among the different athletes I help, the common feedback I hear about Earthing goes something like this: 'I'm sleeping so much better and have less pain. I get up the next day, and I feel so much more recovered. I can't believe the workouts that I'm doing. I should be more tired. My results and improvement are increasing with more frequency. They're staying at a high level. It takes less effort to get and stay where I am.'

"Athletes say frequently they are able to push through the day better. They don't have that midafternoon energy drop. They get up in the morning with much more clarity, ready to seize the opportunity of the day. They seem to need less sleep. They have better quality of sleep. They may have been used to having eight hours of sleep before. Now they need maybe an hour or so less, but they still can perform at the same level. Matter of fact, they even feel better.

"Professional football players live with one degree or another of pain from all the hard physical contact in their sport. They tell me they just don't have the normal pain that they think they should based on what they do. These are the things that I constantly hear.

"Probably the greatest value that I've found with Earthing is that it provides a rock solid biological platform, a basis, for all the other treatments and care that I use. It makes everything else work so much better. Everybody wants a treatment for a specific problem. Earthing, though, is like a universal antidote. It seems to reset the physiological playing field, allowing the body to be its own best healer and do the job it's designed to do —repair and regenerate itself, and create energy to sustain a long and productive life. I think of Earthing as the primer for a canvas on which I paint all the strategies for getting my clients to the top and keeping them there. In art, if you don't properly prime the canvas, the paint won't stick.

"It's now been seven years that I've been Earthing personally and in my work. During that time, there have been only a handful of days that I have not been grounded. On those occasions where for some reason I either forgot my bed pad or the building that I was in didn't allow me to use the technology, I could definitely tell the difference in terms of how I felt and recovered from exercise. I do a lot of traveling, both domestically and internationally, and one of the personal benefits that I found is the dramatic reduction in jet lag. I get up the next day and function fully in the time zone I'm at and not where I came from.

"Earthing is amazingly simple. It's as easy as going barefoot on the beach or in your yard. Or if you have an Earthing device, all you do is plug it in. You lie down, you go to sleep. You do what you normally do. No refills. No prescriptions. No calibrations, settings, timers, no nothing.

"In my view, biology is biology. It doesn't matter who you are. We all share the same basic human biology. What I've observed with high performers in terms of the response to the Earth is exactly what I have observed with patients who aren't athletes. All of us need to perform as best as we can in life and have the stamina to carry out our daily routines, which often are very demanding and stressful. Whatever we can do to enhance our performance and bolster our recovery from day-to-day stresses helps ensure that we become consistent top performers in whatever we do in our lives. That's really what life is all about."

EARTHING AND FOOTBALL

Chike Okeafor, thirty-three, linebacker for the National Football League's Arizona Cardinals: "I've been sleeping grounded regularly for more than five years after experiencing the effect of grounding on a leg injury. It was a hamstring injury in the back of my knee, plus some deep bruising of the thigh, incurred during a practice session. As I lay on a grounded sheet, I watched a computer monitor connected to a real-time thermal imaging camera. I was amazed to see the colors depicting the intensity of the inflammation from the injury cool down quickly, like within fifteen minutes. The intensity was dramatically different within an hour or so. I felt the difference physically, but to see the changes like that so rapidly was mind-blowing.

"I needed to play that weekend in a big game and there wasn't much time to recover. We were thinking it was going to be nothing short of a miracle to get me ready. My naturopath did some work on me, and I slept grounded the rest of that week. I recovered enough to where I was able to play and without injuring myself further. I was sold on grounding from then on.

"There haven't been very many occasions since then that I do not sleep grounded. I can always feel the difference. In those situations, my wife and I always notice that we're not getting as restful sleep as we do when we are grounded. I used to be a guy who needed eight hours of sleep, and I would take ten if I had the opportunity. I quickly saw that with grounding I was well rested with six hours.

"I have also felt a big difference on the days after games. Normally, you are super sore the day after because of the physical nature of the game, from all the hits and banging that goes on. I never ever miss grounding the night after a game because it so dramatically reduces the inflammation. I am not nearly as sore. It feels almost as if I have skipped that tough day of normal recovery. With grounding, the experience is more like how I used to feel on day two after a game."

EARTHING ON THE TRIATHLETE FRONT

Chris Lieto, thirty-seven, a professional triathlete, is three-time Ironman champion and former U.S. National Champion: "I first got involved in the sport more than ten years ago. Early on, I set a goal of being world champion. So I needed to figure out the best route how to get there and as quick as possible. I needed to maximize everything—my effort, my equipment, my supplements, my food, my water, and my recovery process, that is, recovery from injuries and exhaustion, and that's where grounding came in.

"I train full-time. That's my job. I love it. I love being outside and being healthy. My training schedule is a little bit different every day, depending on what race is coming up. The Ironman involves a 2.4-mile swim, followed by a 112-mile bike ride, and then when you're done with all that, you run a marathon. That's 26.2 miles. So it ends up being a very long and tough day to say the least. But that's just in the Ironman. There are also half-Ironman distances, with a 1.2-mile swim, a 56-mile bike race, and a 13.1-mile run, and other variations on the theme as well.

"I usually get in anywhere from three to eight hours of training daily on a regular basis, about twenty to twenty-six hours a week total. That includes swimming and biking four or five days a week and running about five or six days a week. There are days I will rest and not train at all. When I am preparing for an Ironman competition, during the course of a week I'll swim probably twelve miles, bike up to fifteen miles, and build up to about eighty miles a week running.

"The sport is really tough on your body. You have to train so much and for different activities. This is different from most any other sport. For most sports, you go out and train specifically for one event or one thing, and you train for two to four hours a day. Here, you really put your body through the ringer every day. So recovery is a major issue. Anyone can go out and train. But if you don't have that recovery, and your body's not adapting, then the training is just going to be hurting you instead of benefiting you. You have to take the time and the focus to recover. You need to get good sleep and get enough good foods and protein and calories in you. It's vital to stay on top of everything.

"I've been sleeping grounded for more than four years, and it has been a huge boost for me and my recovery process. I'm able to come back a lot stronger and feel a lot better. I noticed right away that I wouldn't get as fatigued on a daily basis. If you're tired and you go out and train, you're just going to dig yourself a hole. I was now able to recover better to be able to workout the next day. Because that's what it's about. You want to get in the workouts day in and day out. But you want to make sure that you recover enough to get that workout to be of benefit. So for me, grounding has been a simple way to recover without really doing anything different.

"The swelling is a lot less. During the day, if I have a chance, I'll put my feet on a grounding pad. When I get done with a workout, I make my recovery food and drink, sit down, and wrap my legs in a recovery bag. Any time for me to be hooked into the Earth is good.

"If I have really sore shin splints or a sore calf or a hurting hip, I'll attach a grounded electrode patch right on the spot. The Earth's energy gets fed straight into that point, and the swelling in that area will go down. Recently, I had an ankle that flared up. For a week, I was applying alternate ice and heat, but it wouldn't go away. I put the patch on it, and the following day it felt normal and I could run that day. So now I use the patch directly on the spot whenever something feels a little sore or is a little swollen. I'll put a patch on and I'm good.

"I haven't won the world championship yet. That's the big goal that has eluded me so far. My career has gotten better and better every year, and even as I am getting older—I'm thirty-seven and racing against guys who are ten years younger—I am keeping up in fitness and my ability to race. Grounding has been a big help in allowing me to do that."

EARTHING AND WEIGHTLIFTING

Ken Jones, Ph.D., fifty-three, Clarksville, Tennessee, is an exercise physiologist, high school math teacher, and football coach. In 2008, he won the American Drug-Free Powerlifting Federation title in the master's 110-kilo division and, later in the year, the World Amateur Athletic Union title: "I've been a powerlifter since the age of twelve, and over the years I've achieved many records with different federations. I have been grounding myself for more than two years, ever since the age of fifty. The most I had squatted before that was 505 pounds. After six months of grounding, I was able to increase my lift to 585 pounds, a jump of 80 pounds. When that happened, at my age, I thought it was a bit strange. So I went to an endocrinologist to find out if something was going on with my testosterone level. He checked me out. My testosterone level was not real high. So that wasn't the thing causing my lifts to go up like I was a kid again.

"I improved across the board. Not just squats, but bench press and dead lifts as well. My overall strength level has gone up. I'm able to lift heavier with the big muscle groups in training and still recover faster than I used to from my workouts. That's a big deal. And then to top things off, I won national and world powerlifting championships last year.

"I didn't change any of my workout patterns. I didn't change my diet. I didn't lay off and then come back. The only thing I can attribute to this unusual improvement is grounding. If I can make those kind of gains at an older age, it should be amazing what someone younger will do."

EARTHING AND GOLF LONGEVITY

Ted Barnett, seventy-one, Palm Desert, California, retired mattress factory owner: "My wife and I owned a mom-and-pop mattress factory. We did at least half the work ourselves and had one or two employees. We made mattresses, delivered them, and set them up in the homes of our customers. In our factory, I was the 'closer.' I ran the big tape-edge machine, which is one of the toughest jobs in a bedding plant. This operation is where you sew the top quilted mattress panel to the side border. People who run this machine for any length of time have problems with their hands because they are constantly pulling hard with their fingers. My hands were in pretty bad shape. I had arthritis, and I was concerned.

"Our factory made some of the first Earthing bed pads for Clint Ober back in 2001 or so. And in the process I got grounded. I thought that grounding might be able to help my hands and my heart. I had had open-heart surgery the year before.

"The grounding helped indeed. My hands stopped hurting. I don't recall exactly how long it took, but I remember that I was significantly impressed to the point that I continued doing it. Even to this day, if I travel or otherwise go without sleeping grounded for two or three days, my hands will start hurting again, as well as the shoulders, neck, and other parts of my body where I have a touch of arthritis. As soon as I get home,

I ground myself. Within one day, or even within hours, I can stop the pain. It disappears.

"I'm an avid golfer and have been so all my life. Now that I'm retired I play practically every day, and even though I'm seventy-one, I'm still very competitive. I was a 2 to 3 handicap golfer in my younger days. Now I'm still at a 4 to 5 handicap level. None of my contemporaries are at my level anymore. All the guys I used to play with when I was younger and who played me even or beat me can't come close to me anymore. They have lost their capacity to play competitively. I have not. I play with the pros my age and I kick their tails. They can't believe it.

"I play golf grounded. I put copper wires in the insole of my shoes, bend them through a hole in the soles, and then bend them again flat against the bottom of the shoes. I think that sleeping and playing grounded has something to do with being supple and able to take the physical beating caused by regular practice and playing. Most people my age stop being competitive on the golf course because they can't take the abuse to their body. They can't practice, swing really hard, or push their games to be a winner because it hurts. So they don't win. They lose. I can't beat the really good twenty- or thirty-year-old kids. Nothing hurts when they swing. But the older ones don't beat me."

CHAPTER 14

The Auto Connection: Earthing on the Move

A truck stop is an unlikely setting for a "scientific" experiment. But one busy truck stop just north of Los Angeles along Interstate 5 was just that for a few days in February 2000. Truckers who stopped there were approached by an enthusiastic trio of Clint Ober and two old friends, Corky and Kathleen Downing.

The three of them were busy enrolling long-haul drivers into a simple experiment. All the drivers had to do was agree to sit on a 10-by-14-inch conductive seat pad connected by a wire to the metal frame under their seat. Installation would take less than five minutes. When they got to their next distant destination, the drivers were asked to write down if they felt any difference while driving with the seat pad, such as any change in tension, pain, or fatigue levels, and then mail in their comments with a provided self-addressed stamped envelope. Any driver doing that would receive a check for $25. And twenty-seven of them, with an average age of forty-eight, did just that. They were all from different parts of the country and didn't know each other.

As Corky explains, "We wanted to test the concept of grounding drivers to the metal frame of their seat, which in turn is connected to the huge metal chassis of the truck. We believed that vehicular grounding in this manner would help ease the strain and tension involved in long-distance driving.

"My wife was the first person to try the seat pad in her car. She didn't like driving at night. It made her nervous and raised her blood pressure.

When she drove sitting on the seat pad, her blood pressure actually went down. She still uses it to this day.

"If you go into any truck stop and examine the counter near the register, you will see a lot of over-the-counter pain pills and no-doze remedies. The truckers live on that stuff. They need them to keep awake and ease their driving aches."

LESS STRESS FOR THE LONG HAUL

Clint Ober was very aware of these common challenges facing long-distance drivers. He had parked in many a truck stop during his years of driving an RV around the country. While living in Ventura in 1999, he thought he could help truckers with a grounded seat pad. So he approached a neighbor who drove up and down California in a big rig. Here's Clint's story:

"I asked to go along with him on one of his trips to test the seat pad. I brought a square of conductive material and put it on his seat, then connected it to the metal frame beneath the seat with an alligator clip. There are 10 tons of metal in a truck like that. Seats in cars and trucks are bolted to the floor, and thus connected to the metal frame of the vehicle. I figured this setup would offer an electrical ground plane that could perhaps serve as a 'sink' into which static electricity from his body could be discharged. A lot of static electricity builds up on the body as a result of the material from the shirt or jacket of a driver or passenger rubbing up and down against the back of the seat as the vehicle is in motion. This phenomenon is called 'triboelectrification,' and it builds up whenever you drive. It's particularly noticeable on dry days whenever you slide across the seat of your car and touch a metal door handle to exit the vehicle after driving a distance. Though sometimes quite jolting, these shocks are not really dangerous to a driver or passenger.

"I took a voltmeter with me on the trip and I measured the trucker's body voltage connected and unconnected. There was a big difference. When the driver was grounded, the buildup on his body disappeared. The electrical potential of the body of the trucker and the truck became the same. The trucker told me at the end the trip that he felt much better and more relaxed than he usually did after his long hauls.

"Based on this experience, I then designed a proper seat pad. It had conductive carbon fibers set into a nylon fabric backed with a soft, non-skid material. We then went out to test it on more truckers."

HAPPY TRUCKERS

Clint, Corky, and Kathleen explained their plan to one of the managers on duty at the busy truck stop north of Los Angeles. She asked to try it first. She lived about three-quarters of an hour from the business and said that she had bad neck pain aggravated by the back-and-forth drive each day. She would have to take pain pills when she arrived at home or at work. After test-driving the seat pad, she said she was convinced. There was no or little pain, and no need for the pills. She gave the "scientists" a green flag to approach the truckers stopping at the station. Their feedback was across-the-board positive. Nearly all of the twenty-seven participants reported more relaxation and reduction in pain and stiffness. Around 70 percent said they experienced less fatigue and more alertness while driving. More than 60 percent said their night vision was improved. Here are some of their individual comments:

- "More alert. Less pain and stiffness." R. M., Federal Way, WA

- "My whole body feels more relaxed." H. S., Brookings, OR

- "Reduction of fatigue." R. N., Lone Pine, CA

- "I've noticed I have fewer aches and pains." R. B., Missoula, MT

- "Stress in shoulders and back is gone." D. C., Houston, TX

- "A great stress and road-rage reliever." R. C., Oklahoma City, OK

- "Helped my headaches go away." R. F. R., Gretna, NE

- "Reduced leg and back pain." C. H., Yakima, WA

As news of the benefits of the seat pad spread throughout the trucking industry, an article in a 2000 publication of the Association of Professional Truck Drivers of America informed its readers that the seat pad addressed the nervous system consequences of extraneous electrical charge on the body resulting from road vibration and the related motion of the driver's body on the vehicle seat. *Overdrive,* a leading publication serving commercial truck owner-operators and company drivers, humorously explained the concept this way: "Lower your stress with honorable discharge."

Over the years, drivers using a conductive seat pad in their vehicles have consistently commented about less tension and fatigue when driving.

CHAPTER 15

The Animal Connection: Earthing and Indoor Pets

Clint Ober recalls an incident from his youth and growing up on a farm in Montana that left a vivid image in his memory: "One day while tending to some cattle with my dad we came upon a calf lying on the ground with a portion of its intestines hanging out of a large gash in its stomach. The mother cow was standing nearby as if protecting the calf. We were not sure what had happened. Maybe dogs or wolves attacked it, or it had gotten tangled up in some barbed wire. My dad took a needle and some coarse thread out of a saddlebag and went over and rolled the calf onto its side. He told me to sit on the calf to hold it still. My dad then pushed the exposed intestines back in the calf's belly and then proceeded to sew her up. No antiseptics. No antibiotics. Upon completion, my dad said she would either live or die and there was nothing more we could do. We were several miles away from the barn. The weather was very cold and it was snowing. There was no way we could have taken the calf back to the barn.

"I didn't think much more about this incident until a week or so later when I saw the same calf running around with the other calves like nothing had happened. Thereafter, I often wondered why outdoor animals seemed to heal up naturally and quickly from wounds as compared to humans, or even indoor pets, who seemed to take much longer to heal and to need excessive treatment and care. So many times I noticed sick animals lying in a dark corner on the Earth and then coming around seemingly healthy again.

"Whenever I asked veterinarians who treated both outdoor and indoor animals about this, they would just shrug and say the outdoor animals are out in Nature and that gives them something that indoor animals don't have. That something obviously includes more sunlight but, as I have learned, the natural healing energy of the Earth. They are connected."

GROUNDED DOGS

Several years ago, pet health writer CJ Puotinen and her husband obtained a grounding bed pad, which improved their sleep. "My husband was a professor of mechanical engineering," she says, "and the theory behind this simple technology made perfect sense to him." A writer of books and magazine articles about holistic pet care, Puotinen wondered whether bed pads could improve the life of animals as well. She contacted Dale Teplitz, a health and energy medicine researcher who had helped conduct several Earthing studies over the years. The two teamed up to design an experiment for dogs in 2007 utilizing a prototype grounded pad.

Together, they identified sixteen canines with histories of unresolved arthritic pain, fatigue, anxiety, hip dysplasia, chronic coughs, old injuries, and emotional problems. For the purpose of the study, the animals slept grounded on the pad for four to six weeks. The owners kept daily and weekly logs of their observations. During the experiment, the animals were only allowed to be naturally grounded for several minutes a day when relieving themselves outdoors.

The typical feedback from owners who kept detailed records included improvements in energy, stamina, flexibility, joint mobility, muscle tone, calmness, sleep, and signs of pain such as limping, stiffness, tentative movements, low activity levels, or a reluctance to jump, play, or move quickly, according to Teplitz.

"After the trial ended, some of the owners stopped using the pads briefly to see if there was any difference in the animals," she added. "They reported seeing pre-trial signs starting to return. That really made them believe in grounding even more."

Chip Feeling Chipper

One participant in the experiment was Chip McGrath, a ten-year-old retired racing Greyhound who belongs to Roberta Mikkelsen of Pearl River, New York. Chip had a bad limp because of joint stress and racing injuries, a result of hard running at speeds up to 45 miles per hour. The dog had also reinjured his leg and was unable to jump onto the couch or into the car for nearly a year.

"Now, thanks to the Earthing pad, he does both all the time," said Mikkelsen. "He has no evidence of pain or joint problems. He's more playful, jumps and runs more, tolerates longer walks, and has far more energy than before. He still limps a bit, but the veterinarian says that's because of the corns on his paws from his earlier racing days."

One of the surprising "side effects" of grounding was an "amazing mental change" in Chip within three weeks of sleeping grounded. "He had always been anxious and afraid of thunder, fireworks, and other loud noises," said Mikkelsen. "He would pant, pace, shake, and hide during storms until the storm was over. Greyhounds who have been raced a lot seem to develop lots of fears, and Chip sure had his share. But that behavior just stopped. The Earthing pad seems to have taken the fear out and calmed him. Now, when the weather is stormy, he is as calm as can be and goes readily off to sleep. For two years in a row now, he has even slept through Fourth of July fireworks."

Impressed by the improvements in her dog, Mikkelsen obtained a bed pad for her husband who suffered with pain from spinal compression fractures. Her husband experienced minor relief, but Mikkelsen was totally surprised about what happened to her own pain problem.

"For two months, my fingers, elbows, hips, and knees had all been hurting, a consequence of overdoing it while laying a brick patio in my backyard," she recalled. "When I got up out of a chair, I could hardly walk. I had to wait a few moments before I could get moving. Within three days of Earthing, my pain disappeared and hasn't returned. I am as spry as before. This was totally unexpected."

Improved Quality—and Length?—of Life

Jill Queen, of Mount Pleasant, North Carolina, has an affinity for rescued standard poodles and two of her older dogs were part of the study. Both animals passed away in 2009, but Queen said that grounding greatly improved their quality of life and probably also extended their lives. Mikey died at fourteen. He had been grounded for nearly two years. Marilyn died at twelve. She had been grounded for a year and a half.

"Most standard poodles tend not to live longer than ten years, so I feel that grounding contributed to a longer life," said Queen.

Mikey's joints were badly affected with degenerative arthritis. He was restless at night. Within one week of grounding, he was showing less signs of stiffness and sleeping better. Improvements continued throughout the trial. At five weeks, he was eager to go for a walk and had more mobility.

"He was doing much better than what his x-rays indicated he could do," Queen said.

Marilyn had a history of arthritis, gastrointestinal problems, lower back disc injuries, pancreatitis, and renal failure. She tended to slip and fall frequently, her paws seeming to come out from under her. She slept restlessly and had poor energy.

Within two weeks of Earthing, her energy level was up. She was more playful and slept better. Her appetite improved. At week three, she was doing more running, less falling, and appeared much steadier on her feet. After five weeks, she was dramatically healthier, calmer, and much more energetic.

One of Queen's observations is that her animals would always seek out the grounded pad to sleep on despite the availability of other, and even more comfortable, doggie beds she had in her house. Wherever she placed the pad, the dogs would look for it.

"They must sense something," she said.

After Mikey and Marilyn died, she obtained another standard poodle. "As soon as the dog entered her home, he went straight for the pad and passed up the other beds. It was amazing to me."

In a report she wrote for the *Whole Dog Journal,* Puotinen observed, "Since time began, animals have lived in direct contact with the Earth. Their feet were always on the ground, they always breathed open air, and the sun and moon illuminated their days and nights. Even after their human companions moved into houses, most dogs lived outdoors. Now people and their pets are indoor creatures. Sure, dogs go for walks and enjoy other outdoor activities, but, like most of us, our dogs often spend more than twenty hours a day inside. If your dog spends most of the day and all of the night indoors, do what you can to increase his time outside. Resting or playing in a fenced yard is perfect, as are long walks, hikes, and swims."

But nothing, she says, makes it as easy to provide the Earth's free electrons to indoor pets as an Earthing pad. "In addition to receiving reports from dog owners about how their companions' arthritis symptoms and other physical problems improve, I have heard from several people whose dogs and cats take turns sleeping on the grounded pad. When my Labrador retriever received her bed pad, it wasn't long before Pumpkin, my husband's red tabby cat, was taking naps on it. Neither of these animals have any health problems, so I haven't noticed a difference in symptoms or behavior, but I think it's interesting that they are both so drawn to the mat."

THE GROUNDED COCKATOO

Don Scott is an aviculturist in Escondido, California. He is the founder of The Chloe Sanctuary, a rescue shelter for cockatoos and parrots. He finds "foster" homes for the birds and trains people how to handle them as pets.

His experience with Chloe, the namesake of his sanctuary, suggests that the use of a grounded perch may help prevent or minimize the common psychoses—screaming, pacing, biting, and feather destructive behavior—of caged birds.

"Something substantial changed after I installed a grounded perch in Chloe's cage," he said. That was in mid-2008. Chloe was a twenty-five-year-old umbrella cockatoo at the time. She had been rescued from previous owners unable to give her proper care.

When Chloe came into Scott's care in 2003, she had an established problem of feather-destructive behavior due to being left alone for weekends at a time. According to veterinary records, Chloe had apparently been doing this since 2000. Social birds like these do not do well in situations of sustained separation from those they consider their flock. Cockatoos mate for life and always remain within screeching distance of their mate except when caring for their young. This devotion applies to their human "mates" as well.

"Chloe has become much calmer with the grounded perch," according to Scott. "She used to intensely pull out her feathers. It was bad. She doesn't do that anymore. She may tug at her feathers a little bit now and then, but only at the tips and not at the base as she used to do.

"Before, she would sit a good deal of the time in the cage and show little interest in her environment. Now she forages more for food and plays more with her toys. She is more active and playful."

The perch consists of an 18-inch stainless steel bathroom grab bar that Mr. Scott bought at Home Depot. He mounted it on a 1-by-3-inch piece of pine, attached a copper wire and connected it to the ground terminal in a wall outlet.

The grounded perch is not the highest perch in the cage. It's in the middle. Birds prefer a high perch at night out of an instinct for safety. The higher the perch the less chance of being attacked.

"But Chloe prefers this lower perch and uses it consistently at night," said Scott. "Instinctively, she picked up something that attracted her. What's fascinating is that once the grounded perch became disconnected and I wasn't aware of it, Chloe immediately sensed some difference and ignored the perch and went back to the perch at the higher level. I wondered why this was happening and then I discovered the disconnection. After reconnecting, Chloe went back to sitting on the middle perch again."

Scott said that Chloe was initially upset by the new perch but quickly felt very comfortable on it, and without screaming to be let out of the cage. Since installing the perch, she stopped walking a "figure eight" repeated pattern on the cage door, another sign of wanting to get out.

CHAPTER 16

The Future Connection: The Earthing Revolution Ahead

This book is a statement about Nature and health. Health is natural, and part of being naturally healthy and functioning optimally appears to involve connectedness to the Earth. Being disconnected seems to be both unnatural and unhealthy. The disconnect creates unnecessary suffering in the form of sickness, inflammation, pain, and poor sleep—the consequences of an electron deficiency. Connecting to the Earth remedies that deficiency and its consequences.

We think this book offers a relevant piece of the answer to T. H. Huxley's prodigious question about determining our place in Nature and our relationship to the cosmos. We live on our planet. But we have insulated ourselves from it—and at great cost. As a society, we are hurting and unhealthy, and we have been that way for quite a while. The health statistics indicate that we are no longer the hardy, red-blooded folks we used to be. We stress our bodies to the breaking point. We eat the wrong foods and don't exercise.

Back fifty years ago or so, with the emergence of medical insurance plans, people expected they'd be taken care of when they got old and there would be a pill for every illness. Today, there is a pill for practically every illness, but the pills don't particularly cure anything or make us healthier.

The late John Knowles, M.D., head of the Massachusetts General Hospital and the Rockefeller Foundation during the 1960s and 1970s, put it this way years ago: "People have been led to believe that national health insurance, more doctors, and greater use of high-cost, hospital-based technologies will improve health. Unfortunately, none of them will."

At the time, politicians and doctors had become increasingly concerned about the rising costs of health care. Sound familiar? Such costs were eating up about 8 percent of the domestic national product back then. Today, the percentage has more than doubled and is supposed to reach 20 percent in a few years! Politicians and doctors are still concerned, but concern hasn't helped much.

And the future?

Ouch! It hurts to look ahead.

HEALTH CARE CHANGE . . . FROM THE GROUND UP

Nearly 80 million American baby boomers will soon turn sixty-five, and as they do, there will obviously be more people with chronic diseases and higher medical care costs draining an already strained medical system. Without any significant changes, the surge may break the Medicare coffers—and predictions for that have already surfaced.

The Council of State Governments, a leading multi-branch organization forecasting policy trends, said in a 2006 alert on chronic disease that along with more forecasted disease among the older population, there is also the issue of more children entering their teen years, college, and adulthood with diabetes, high blood pressure, and other effects of overweight, physical inactivity, and unhealthful eating. "Some experts estimate that the generation growing up today will be the first to live a shorter life than their parents and grandparents. This will have a tremendous effect on public resources and the ability of public agencies to provide health care and social services, while draining a critical U.S. resource—the work force."

The status quo isn't working. The situation threatens the health of individuals, the family, and nations everywhere. Declining health is hardly an American monopoly. The health of all humanity is in crisis. The many ailments besetting the United States are symptomatic of a planetary catastrophe in the making before our eyes and headlined in the news every single day.

The analogy of raising cows may be appropriate here. If humans were cows, they would have to be taken out and shot. Who could afford the vet bill?

Health care, as it operates today, is impotent, exorbitant, and ineffective. Chronic disorders are out of control, and the solution is really not in the hands of government or insurers. It is in our hands. Our health, or lack of it, is by and large the result of how we live.

"Self-care is the only effective way to ensure good health and a longer, fuller life," wrote Joseph D. Beasley, M.D., and Jerry J. Swift, M.A., in an epic 1989 Ford Foundation book, *The Kellogg Report: The Impact of Nutrition, Environment & Lifestyle on the Health of Americans* (Bard College). "While there is a crying need for reforms of the health care system, the most needed reform of all is in our own attitudes—we patients must become activists for our own health."

These and many other similar admonitions have largely remained beyond the hearing range of most people, who persist in overeating unnatural food and avoiding physical activity. So we just become sicker and sicker.

Instead of focusing on health insurance, we need to emphasize health assurance. We reach that greater level of protection by removing the major sources of stress and toxicity in our lives. In this book, we propose one surprisingly and utterly simple means of helping to reach that goal.

EARTHING'S PARADIGM-CHANGING HEALTH AND ECONOMIC POTENTIAL

Earthing represents a discovery of the first magnitude, as potentially significant and globally sweeping as electricity, telephones, radio, television, and computers. Consider the changes that new technologies like these brought to society in their time. We are still riding the waves of innovation they generated in terms of jobs and economies. Earthing, like these concepts, is disruptive in that it changes how people live. It is something evolutionary and, at the same time, revolutionary.

We believe that Earthing can change the way medicine itself is practiced, adding major effectiveness in healing while lowering the cost of treatments for many diseases. Keep in mind that the physiology of the grounded person appears to be different—in a more efficient and healthier way—than that of an ungrounded person.

As more research rolls out, we envision Earthing units being installed in spas and the clinics of health practitioners. We envision patients being

grounded in hospitals and nursing homes. Sophisticated electrically operated equipment and instrumentation are grounded in medical and health
care facilities. The beds are grounded. Why not the patients in those beds?

Looking ahead, we believe that Earthing can generate a broad societal
and economic overhaul.

Economies are based on businesses that create profits, jobs, and wealth.
We think that Earthing offers a huge bonanza for business the world over.
Earthing has the potential to benefit—and change—the world in many
ways. It is equally available to the richest and the poorest, to both the
industrialized and the developing world.

Earthing will affect all society—literally from the ground up, starting
with the shoe industry. The simple insertion of a few cents of conductive
carbon or some other similar material in the soles of shoes can bring people into contact again with the Earth's healing energy. The shoe manufacturing industry hasn't acted in bad faith, but its innovations have
contributed to the rise of chronic illness. Here's a golden opportunity for
the shoe industry to redeem and reinvent itself in the name of health . . .
and expanded sales. What a glorious prospect! Every year a person buys
at least one new pair of shoes. For a small investment on the part of the
industry, so much good can be done in the marketplace. As a consumer,
start asking about grounded shoes the next time you make a purchase.
Create the demand.

Earthing has the potential to thoroughly revolutionize the bedding and
mattress industry. Every eight years on average, people replace their mattresses in the United States. About 30 million are sold each year. And there
is a mattress store for every 20,000 homes in America. Here is an industry that sells comfort in all forms: water, air, springs, foam, latex. But just
by adding a few dollars' worth of conductive material to the mattress and
connecting it to the Earth, it can improve the health of a society full of
insomniacs while it sleeps. The new mattress bottom line will be: more
comfort, better sleep, less pain, better health.

Imagine the rush to buy grounded mattresses!

Hotels have been spending billions on twenty-first century upgrades
such as flat-screen TVs, wireless Internet, trendier bars, and fancier show-
ers. Imagine the appeal of hotels offering weary travelers grounded mattresses to promote sleep and elimination of jet lag.

The shoe and mattress industry have blockbuster products to sell and, while they are at it, become a part of the health care industry. These are the best place to start the Earthing revolution. Is there any simpler kind of health reform than that? When you go out to purchase shoes and mattresses, you will simultaneously be buying better health for yourself.

There are innumerable business opportunities to bring the Earth's healing electrons up into our lives so that everyone lives grounded most of each and every day. Homes, offices, and schools need to be grounded. That includes floors, carpets, and furniture. Even cars can get a modified dose of grounding with a simple seat pad. All these basic parts of society's infrastructure can be inexpensively outfitted with conductive material, creating a whole Earthing industry to ground new and existing houses. Out of this will come whole new manufacturing, marketing, distributing, and installation industries, just like exists today with telephone or cable systems.

Think of how all this will impact the way we design our living and working environments. Can you imagine what effect all this will have on the health statistics we cited above? And on the economy of the world in terms of new jobs, careers, research, products, education, services, and even tax revenue for cash-strapped governments? For corporations, just think of what this will do to their own health insurance premiums and cost of doing business. Instead of a malignant cycle of bad health, we can create a benign cycle of good health that embraces and benefits both employers and employees alike.

Earthing is the future. Humanity needs to reconnect to the planet, to our natural electrical state, and to our natural state of good health.

It's so simple to do.

Our book is a bugle call. Wake up, people. Go out. Ground yourself. Reintroduce your bare feet to the ground. Sleep grounded, and, if you can, work grounded, play grounded, and watch TV grounded.

If you haven't done it by now, go sit or stand barefoot outside (weather permitting) for a half hour or so. If you have pain, see what difference it makes. Then ask yourself if reconnecting with the Earth might be the most amazing health discovery *you* have ever made.

We think that reconnecting with the Earth is amazing, and may, in fact, be *the* most important health discovery ever.

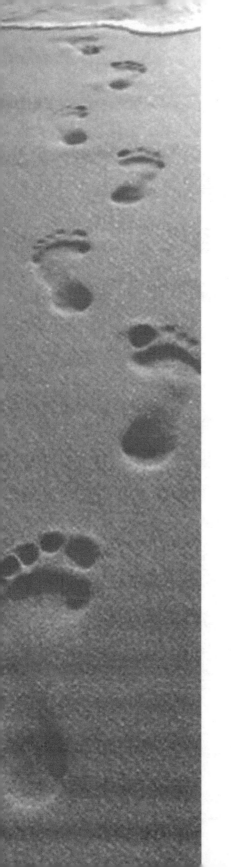

Appendices

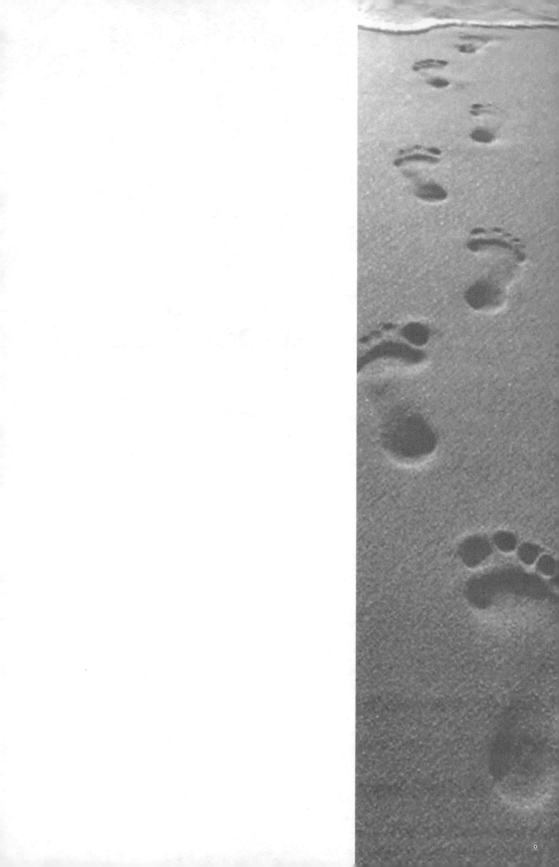

Technical Notes on Grounding and Earthing Methods

Physicists and electrical engineers have chosen the Earth as the most obvious "ground," or reference point, for all electrical power grids. The Earth provides a reference voltage, that is, the ground or zero potential against which all other voltages are established and measured. There is no absolute electric potential. What is measured is the difference in electric potential between two points—one being the Earth, the reference point.

What Exactly Is a Ground?

A ground is defined as a conductive object that makes a direct electrical connection to Earth and has the ability to absorb or dissipate an electrical charge, thereby maintaining a grounded object at the stable electrical potential of the Earth. Grounding is central to the safe and stable usage of electricity. A ground connection serves as an electrical "sink" that minimizes the susceptibility of electromagnetic interference in communication systems; reduces the risk of equipment damage due to lightning; eliminates electrostatic buildup, which can damage system components; and helps protect people who service and repair electrical, electronic, and computer equipment.

In effect, an electrical ground drains away any unwanted buildup of electrical charge. When a device or person is connected to an Earth ground, that device or person will equalize with, and maintain, the stable electrical potential of the Earth.

An "Earth ground" usually consists of a ground rod driven into the

Earth. In a car, truck, aircraft, or a spacecraft, there is no such thing as a true Earth ground. But if the mass of metal comprising the vehicle is substantial, that mass can simulate an Earth ground reasonably well.

Earthing Methods and Considerations

We expect that after reading this book many people will want to experiment with Earthing in order to experience the effects that Earthing may have on their health and sleep.

The easiest method, of course, is as simple as routinely going outdoors and placing your bare feet directly on the Earth for thirty minutes at a time. But being barefoot is not always an option.

We have described a variety of personal Earthing methods in the book that we call "barefoot substitutes." They involve use of a ground rod or a specially designed wall plug that can be connected to conductive floor mats, chair pads, sheets, mattresses, and common electrode patches to Earth individuals indoors while sleeping or sitting. We have even mentioned grounded shoes.

Few of these systems are now commercially available, but we expect more to become accessible in the near future. Keep in mind that most of these systems were developed primarily for use in proof-of-concept Earthing studies. Ways were needed to Earth people for study purposes when they were confined to one place during a testing period. From the start, many study participants and researchers requested sample Earthing devices for friends and families, leading to further development and testing of various Earthing product forms for indoor home use. Some proved to be functional and effective. Others, less so.

The primary concern in developing these home/office systems was to ensure both effectiveness and safety. The systems used in the studies consisted of a ground rod placed directly in the Earth, along with a fuse-protected ground wire to connect the Earthing test device to the ground rod. (See Figure A-1.) When home grounding systems were given to individuals who requested sample devices, we recommended that an electrician or professional cable installer be employed to install the ground system, which included placing of the ground rod, running the ground wire, and mounting a permanent wall outlet for easy connection of Earthing devices.

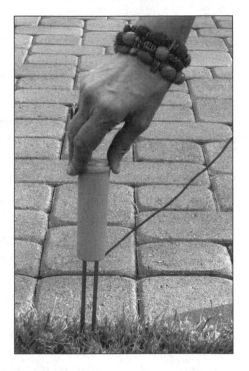

Figure A-1.
Placing ground rod in Earth.

Most people just ran the ground wire out a window and set the ground rod themselves as a temporary installation until they could arrange a permanent installation. Some just left it there where it was initially placed without a problem. People were always cautioned to use a location where the rod and the wire would not present a tripping hazard.

In developing and testing home Earthing systems, the following facts have become clear:

1. The most effective Earthing system in the studies consisted of a ground rod placed directly in the Earth with a ground wire running into the home and connected directly to the Earthing device (sheet, floor pad, etc). Still, most people who use electrical ground systems (that is, plugged into a properly grounded wall outlet in their home or office) report similar health benefits to those using dedicated Earth ground systems. For best results, it is prudent to test the outlet for proper grounding or have a professional grounding technician/electrician check your electrical ground system before use as a method of personal Earthing.

2. For safety reasons, the ground wire must be insulated and contain an in-line 2mA fuse or current-limiting resistor of similar value for protection from an accidental electrical event. It is unlikely that such an event would occur in a typical home environment because all modern electrical appliances and devices are protected with polarized cords and are made to conform with UL (North American) and CE (European) safety standards.

3. Many individuals have experimented with common personal electro-static discharge (ESD) grounding systems for Earthing. These systems are used in the electronics industry and are designed to prevent the buildup of static electricity on the body, which could otherwise damage the microchips and hardware that employees handle when building or repairing computers and electronic equipment. Such ESD grounding devices are generally connected to the third-prong ground port of an electrical outlet. In factories where employees use EDS grounding systems, an electrical engineer or electrician will test and verify that the electrical ground is in good working order before allowing employees to connect themselves to this system.

Our testing of ESD grounding systems failed to totally reproduce the same effects as in our studies where we used a direct Earth ground system. This difference was due to the dampening effect on the Earth ground signal by the in-line 1 megohm resistor that all ESD ground cords contain.

4. Many individuals who learn about the health effects of Earthing ask how they can make their own system for use at home. Some, and especially those who live in apartments and high-rise buildings, ask if they can use the electrical ground system in their building for Earthing. From our experience, the electrical ground system in a building—that is, the use of wall outlets—is the only option that most people living in multi-story buildings will have, unless they can drop a long wire out the window and connect it to a ground rod in the Earth below.

In general, a house or building electrical ground system will work for Earthing, as all electrical ground systems are connected directly to a ground rod driven into the Earth. However, there are certain problems that may exist with these systems:

- Most residential homes built in the United States before the 1960s do not have an electrical ground system. Many of these homes have recently been remodeled with the old-style outlets being replaced with newer fixtures containing a ground port. In appearance, it may look as if the home has an electrical ground system, but there is usually no ground wire connected to the newer ground port outlets. Often, there is no ground wire in the walls to connect to the ground port. Thus, in many older homes there is no ground system. In these cases, use of a dedicated Earth ground rod system is the only option.

- Some home electrical outlets are miswired. The most common wiring error is that of the ground and neutral being reversed. In order to verify that electrical ground outlets are correctly wired, inexpensive outlet-wiring checkers are available at all hardware and electrical retail outlets. Always check the outlet-wiring configuration before using an electrical ground for Earthing.

- Many electrical ground systems are prone to carry induced high-frequency electrical "noise" emitted by electrical appliances and motors running in the home. The noise also radiates from appliances into the general living environment as electromagnetic fields (EMFs). To verify the level of electrical noise in your living environment or on your electrical ground system requires an electrical engineer or specially trained electrician to take measurements with an oscilloscope grounded to an independent Earth ground. Even with such electrical noise, use of an electrical ground system for Earthing is safe with the use of an Earthing system designed specifically for personal grounding. It is the potential disturbance that electrical noise may have on the nervous system of an electrically sensitive individual that is an issue with the use of home electrical ground systems. For such people, the best Earthing option is to bypass the electrical system inside the house and connect to a dedicated outside ground rod. Moreover, such systems have an in-line resistor that prevents any harmful flow of current, such as could occur from accidental contact with a live electrical wire or a shorted appliance.

Lightning

One of the most common technical questions asked about Earthing is: Do I have to worry about lightning if I am grounded to the Earth?

Lightning is a massive natural phenomenon that is unpredictable and challenging to totally protect against. It is poorly understood. The following will help you understand how and usually when lightning occurs and what is your likelihood of being hit when grounded to the Earth.

Most lightning strikes occur in the summer during the afternoon (70 percent between noon and 6:00 p.m.). As the air temperature warms, evaporation increases. The warm moist air rises and forms fluffy cumulus clouds. As the moisture accumulates, the clouds darken and change into cumulonimbus or thunderstorm clouds with a flattened base and puffy top reaching as high as 40,000 feet. The upper portion of a thunderstorm cloud develops a positive electrical charge, and the bottom of the cloud develops a negative charge. Negative charges repel negative charges and attract positive charges. So, as the thundercloud passes overhead, a concentration of positive charges accumulates in and on all conductive objects below the cloud. Since negative charges closer to the clouds are most efficiently repelled by the negative charges of the cloud, positive charges tend to accumulate at the top of the highest objects on the ground. In most cases that means high ground, trees, communication towers, and aerial power, telephone, and cable TV lines. It could also be you—if you are standing out in the open and are the tallest object in the area. Example: you are out playing golf and standing in the middle of the fairway.

Homes are rarely hit by lightning. When it does occur, the lightning most often takes the path of least resistance to the ground. Generally, the path of least resistance to ground in a home would include large conductive systems like the plumbing pipes, electrical wiring network, or telephone and cable TV lines, all of which are directly grounded to the Earth.

The National Safety Council reports that your odds of dying from a lightning strike in one year are 1 in 6 million (www.nsc.org/research/odds. aspx). To put this in perspective, your odds of being hit and killed by an automobile as a pedestrian in the same period are 1 in fifty thousand—a risk 120 times greater. This information suggests that being hit by lightning is rather unlikely. However, follow standard lightning safety guidelines as directed by National Weather Service (www.lightningsafety.noaa. gov) if you live in a lightning-prone area. Disconnect your Earthing device and don't use it during lightning and thunderstorms.

The Physics of Earthing: A Discussion on Current Understanding

Gaetan Chevalier, Ph.D.,
Visiting Scientist, Developmental and Cell Biology Department,
University of California at Irvine

The Earth is the most negatively charged entity in the immediate human environment. As you lift off the surface and gain altitude, the electric potential increases by about 200 volts with every meter (200 V/m). This is a little known but well-established scientific fact. At several kilometers of altitude, the vertical atmospheric voltage increase begins to slow. As you go higher, the increase shrinks to 150 and then 100 volts per meter. At around 100 kilometers, the increase stops.

In fair weather, when the sky is blue and there are little or no clouds, the electric potential difference is 250,000 to 500,000 volts between the upper part of the atmosphere (called the ionosphere because it is ionized and so conducting) and the Earth's surface. Visualize this system as two conductors, one at zero volts (the ground) and the other at 250,000 to 500,000 volts at an altitude of about 100 kilometers (62.5 miles).

Fair weather atmosphere is not a good conductor (especially close to the ground), but it is not a perfect insulating medium either. There is a very small current of electrons escaping the ground at a rate of about 1 microamp per square kilometer (approximately equivalent to a power loss of 1 microwatt per square meter). This is called the fair weather current, a component of an immense natural phenomenon known as the "global electrical circuit" (see Figure B-1 on the following page).

The global circuit is primarily recharged by cumulonimbus clouds. During

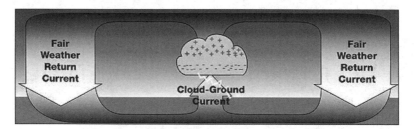

Figure B-1. Global electrical circuit. A current coming up from the ground at the location of lightning (depositing electrons into the earth) and returning to the ground elsewhere. *Source:* NASA/MSFC (Dooling)

an active thunderstorm, the collection of clouds in the storm generates an average current of about 1 amp down to the surface of the Earth. There are an estimated 1,000 to 2,000 thunderstorms happening globally at any one time, and collectively these storms produce as many as 5,000 lightning strikes per minute. Thus, an electrical current of 1,000 to 2,000 amps is continually transferring a negative charge to the surface of the Earth and an equal and opposite charge to the upper atmosphere. The electrical charge continually flowing into the ionosphere from the cumulonimbus clouds maintains the fair weather current flowing to the surface.

Suppose a dust particle floats in the atmosphere at about two meters above ground (about six foot five, the height of a tall human). The electric potential at that level is 400 volts. The particle will acquire a positive electric charge (from collisions with surrounding atmospheric particles) and maintain its electric potential at 400 volts. If the particle rises to four meters it will acquire an electric charge that maintains its electric potential at 800 volts. Whatever the height, the electrical charge of the particle adopts the potential existing at that specific level.

Imagine yourself as that tall individual and you are wearing running shoes. Your feet will be less than an inch above ground and your head would be located at an atmospheric level with an electric potential of about 400 volts. Since you are a conductor, your electric potential will be an average of the electric potential at the ground level and that at 2 meters: about 200 volts (with a current continuously flowing on the surface of your body from head to foot). If you live on the second floor of an apartment complex at about 4 meters above ground, even if not wearing your running shoes but on a wooden floor, then your feet are now planted at an atmospheric level where the electric potential is 800 volts and your head at an electric potential of 1,200 volts, an average electric potential of 1,000 volts on your body! That's not a small level. The higher you live off the ground, the higher your electric potential compared to the ground.

"The High Life"—A Voltage/Grounding/Health Connection?

Is it possible to relate the "high life"—in altitude terms—to a health risk? Is our health being compromised by living and working in high rises?

One recent study conducted at the University of Iowa monitored seniors over a twelve-year period and found a surprising 40 percent higher risk of stroke among those living in multi-story residences compared to ground-floor houses. The revelation was the most striking among a handful of more conventional associations linked to stroke risks in an elderly population following hospitalization for a variety of health issues. The researchers suggested that multi-story living could be related to "greater physical, social and psychological burdens faced by older adults in these settings." We wonder if living at a higher electrical potential of several hundred or more volts, along with the lack of immediate ground, might create a significant electron deficiency in the body and have a pronounced effect on health. Something to think about.

Something else to think about is a recently published analysis in the journal *Cancer* indicating that people living in urban areas are more likely to develop late-stage cancer than those residing in suburban and rural areas. The researchers, using data from the Illinois State Cancer Registry, set out to investigate the rural and urban differences in late-stage diagnoses of breast, colorectal, lung, and prostate tumors—the four major types of cancer. They found that for colorectal and prostate cancers, and to a lesser extent breast cancer, the disparities stemmed from a higher concentration of more vulnerable and economically disadvantaged populations in Chicago and its suburbs. A lower rate of late-stage diagnosis in rural areas reflected a greater prevalence of elderly patients who frequent doctors more often and undergo more age-related cancer screenings. However, these differences could not explain the geographic disparity for lung cancer. In the cities and high-rise buildings, the electrically sensitive lungs breathe in more positively charged air particles. The lungs are not only a target in terms of conventional pollution, but in the presence of an electron deficiency (lack of grounding) the higher density of positively charged particles may create more oxidative stress and free radicals than down at the first-story level.

Yet another factor to ponder here is the combination of a lack of grounding and increased positive charge in the air as an unrecognized cause of the so-called sick building syndrome. According to the U.S. Environmental Protection Agency (EPA), "sick buildings" refer to situations in which building occupants experience acute health and discomfort effects that appear "linked to time spent in a building, but no specific illness or cause can be identified. The complaints may be localized in a particular room or zone, or may be widespread throughout the building."

Experts don't know the causes. They suggest concerns such as inadequate ventilation, chemical contaminants from indoor and outdoor sources, and biological contaminants. "These elements may act in combination, and may supplement other complaints such as inadequate temperature, humidity, or lighting. Even after a building investigation, however, the specific causes of the complaints may remain unknown."

The possibility of an Earthing connection should be investigated. As was discussed in Chapter 7, experts have raised the issue of health risks from man-made electromagnetic environments in office settings and cited lack of grounding as a contributing factor, referring to evidence produced by Earthing research. When you add to this the element of increased positive charge density with height, we may be dealing indeed with a powerful combination of unheralded issues conspiring to undermine health, energy, and performance. Keep in mind that electromagnetic fields (EMFs) are AC (they vary with time). They are composed of electric and magnetic fields artificially produced by humans. The 200 V/m is a DC (static) electric field only and a natural phenomenon that has existed for eons. EMF and 200 V/m are separate entities and should not be confused with each other.

The EMF Connection

Now imagine that you are grounded. If your body is somehow coupled to the Earth, no matter where you are, you are at the electric potential of the ground. That means all of you, from head to foot. Your electric potential is zero and no positive charge can charge you up. You are a part of the ground. You are shielded from whatever happens in the atmosphere. If positive charges are present in your environment and "stick to you," the Earth will provide the electrons to cancel the positive charges and maintain your electric potential at the same level as it is: zero volts. If EMFs hit your body, their effect is cancelled by the electrons within your body supplied by the ground. Nothing can change your electric potential, except uncoupling yourself from the Earth.

Being grounded means your body's internal organs are shielded from any electrostatic or electromagnetic interference in the atmosphere. This provides for a very quiet electrical "milieu" inside the body where no external electric or magnetic fields can disrupt the internal functions maintaining homeostasis and health. This includes digestion, internal repairs, wound healing, and all metabolic activities. Keep in mind that all chemical or biochemical reactions are electrical in nature and so are susceptible to being disturbed by external electric and magnetic fields. Grounding prevents these disturbances. This is how living beings evolved on the Earth!

Grounding also provides a reference point for all electrical activities of the body. Any electrical appliance needs a ground, a reference point, to define the values of the voltages inside its electronic circuits. Even sophisticated equipment such as digital-storage oscilloscopes cannot function properly without a clear reference point. Without it, all the voltages inside the appliance are ill defined and the electronic circuits, which are designed to work based on a reference point, cannot operate correctly. They give random voltage values. This situation can damage expensive equipment.

The human body is by far the most complex piece of "equipment" on the planet. It has evolved in contact with the Earth. All its internal processes are just like electronic circuits. They are all based on bioelectrical processes that need a defined ground to operate well. The body, being so complex, has developed internal mechanisms to help it cope with a temporary disconnect from the Earth, but in the long run the lack of connection takes its toll. Eventually, the body will lose its reference point (even the one that it made for itself temporarily). This results in internal functions becoming increasingly out of sync not only with the Earth but also with each other. For example, the body loses the ability to recognize what is "self" and what is "not self," and thus starts an autoimmune attack on its own cells.

EMFs are ubiquitous, and we live immersed in the invisible traffic of these chaotic fields. Their potential for creating internal interference in the body, as was noted earlier in the book, varies from person to person and in different locations, depending on the intensity and frequencies of the fields.

EMFs occupy such a vast spectrum of frequencies (from 0 to 1,000,000,000,000,000,000,000 Hz or 10^{21} Hz) that they need to be grouped in different frequency bands in order to determine their health effects on humans. One such grouping of frequencies has been created by the European Commission's independent Scientific Committee on Emerging and Newly Identified Health Risks (SCENIHR). This committee divided the spectrum into four frequency bands:

1. Radio frequency (RF) (100 kHz < f ≤ 300 GHz)

2. Intermediate frequency (IF) (300 Hz < f ≤ 100 kHz)

3. Extremely low frequency (ELF) (0 < f ≤ 300 Hz)

4. Static (0 Hz)

Frequencies higher than 300 GHz were not considered by the commission because their mechanisms for affecting human beings are well known and entirely different from lower frequency bands. These higher frequency bands include (in order of increasing frequencies): infrared light (IR), visible light, ultraviolet (UV) light, x-rays, and gamma (gamma) rays. I will limit the discussion here to the extremely low frequency, or ELF, band, the most studied band and with the most commonly encountered frequencies.

In 2007, SCENIHR reported finding no clear evidence of an effect in bands other than the ELF band for lack of good epidemiological studies. The committee's report concluded that ELF magnetic fields are possibly carcinogenic, chiefly based on childhood leukemia data. There is, however, no generally accepted mechanism to explain how ELF magnetic field exposure may cause leukemia. For breast cancer and cardiovascular disease, recent research has indicated that an association is unlikely, while for neurodegenerative diseases and brain tumors, the link to ELF fields remains uncertain. A relation between ELF fields and symptoms (sometimes referred to as electromagnetic hypersensitivity) has not been demonstrated.

Electromagnetic fields, as the name implies, are comprised of electric and magnetic fields. These fields are related but have very different effects. Electric fields are generated by electric charges (protons and electrons) even when there is no motion. Magnetic fields exist only when charges are in motion. For example, the magnetic field of a magnet is generated by the electrons of the magnetic metal spinning around the nucleus of their atom in the same way and in the same direction. They are all aligned. Their correlated rotational movement around their respective nucleus creates a magnetic field. Any electron spinning around any atom produces a magnetic field but in many substances—wood, plastic, rubber, and all insulating materials—they are not aligned. Their alignment is random due to other internal forces and so there is no net magnetic field that we can feel. If an electric charge is at rest in a magnetic field, the magnetic field will have no effect on the charge. When the charge is in motion, the magnetic field will make it rotate around an imaginary point. An electric field, in contrast, will always make electrical charges move in the direction of the field (for positive charges) or in the direction opposite to the field (for negative charges). In all materials, positive charges are in the nucleus. The nucleus cannot move or the substance would be destroyed. So in most practical applications, it is the electrons that move.

If you have followed this discussion closely you have probably deduced that since a change in motion implies an electric field that is changing, we have to conclude that a changing electric field will produce a magnetic field. The opposite is also true; a varying magnetic field produces an electric field, and that is why an electromagnetic field can propagate in space. The varying electric field produces a magnetic field, which produces an electric field, which produces a magnetic field, and this process repeats and goes on indefinitely in space and time. Motors work on the same principle that a current (electric charges in motion) produces a magnetic field, which acts on magnets placed on the rotor, which in turn makes the motor rotate.

Within an ungrounded body, electrons and other charged particles react mainly to the electric field component of the electromagnetic fields present in the immediate environment. Because their movement within the body is very slow, they do not respond well to magnetic fields. Internal electrons close to the surface of the skin are the most susceptible to perturbation, and EMFs at 60 Hz (and its harmonics, 120 Hz, 180 Hz, 240 Hz, and higher multiples of 60 Hz) are believed to have very little penetration power into the skin. The electric field is stopped by surface charges. However, the magnetic field penetrates the body very deeply and will produce electric fields inside the body. At 60 Hz, EMF energy is 10 billion times smaller than that needed to break even the weakest chemical bond. Still, there are known mechanisms by which 60 Hz electric and magnetic fields could produce biological effects without breaking chemical bonds. The 60 Hz electric fields can exert forces on charged and uncharged molecules or cellular structures within tissues. These forces can cause movement of charged particles, orient or deform cellular structures, orient dipolar molecules, or induce voltages across cell membranes. The magnetic fields at 60 Hz can exert forces on cellular structures, but since biological materials are largely nonmagnetic (they do not have a net magnetic field like a magnet has) these forces are usually very weak.

The present understanding of the scientific community on power-frequency (60 Hz) fields can summarized as follows:

- Exposure to these fields cannot be proven to be absolutely safe.

- A relationship has been established between residential and occupational exposure to these fields and human health hazards (including cancer).

- If there is a human health hazard, it is very small or it is restricted to small subgroups (such as young people and leukemia); the possibility of a large and general hazard has been ruled out.

It is my belief that the last consensus statement will be proven wrong scientifically through Earthing research and other future research. Even though no study has been conclusive so far, we have seen that some individuals are indeed ultra-sensitive and can be severely affected. "Electrical hypersensitivity" cannot be explained by any known mechanisms, as the threshold for known interactions are at least fifty times higher than actual exposures levels. Nevertheless, this hypersensitivity is a real phenomenon (two such cases were described in Chapter 10) and may develop as a result of loss of connection to the Earth.

The Body's Internal Clock

For any organism to function properly, it must control the timing of its biological functions. That is why all higher organisms, from plants to insects, reptiles, birds and mammals, and even some lower unicellular forms of life such as bacteria, have developed an internal biological clock over millions of years. In humans, the master clock of all the body's bio-logical clocks is located in the suprachiasmatic nucleus of the hypothala-mus, as we have already mentioned. The alternating day and night mode of Earth's cycle is so reliable that living beings adjust their behavior and physiology according to its rhythm. The timing of many daily processes such as foraging, feeding, or rest can be determined or modulated by the endogenous circadian clock. Scientists consider that the major *zeitgeber* (German for time-giver or synchronizer) of the internal clock is the light from the periodically occurring light-dark cycle. Earthing experiments have shown that it is not the only zeitgeber. People who travel great distances have repeatedly reported that grounding for half an hour after arrival sig-nificantly reduces, if not completely eliminates, jet lag. This phenomenon is best explained by the body sensing different frequencies from the elec-trons of the Earth and receiving "local cues" from these vibrating electrons as to time of day. Further research is needed to prove this effect, but anec-dotal evidences accumulated over the years are strong enough for this effect to deserve mention.

Ground as a Biological Power Source

These fluctuating electrons also carry energy. The energy is provided by the global electrical circuit, a complex system involving the Earth, the atmosphere, and the sun. The Earthing experiments and anecdotal expe-riences suggest there might be a power component to being grounded. Just like an appliance receives power when plugged into a power outlet, the human body may receive power from the Earth when grounded. Tes-timonials presented in this book suggest that people feel "energized" when grounded. Earthing studies suggest that the body starts a healing process after twenty to thirty minutes or so of grounding, an indication the body feels that it has more energy.

Earthing, Inflammation, and Healing

Observations and feedback from many Earthers over the years suggest a mechanism by which the "electron infusion" from Earthing helps the body stay healthy, recover from illnesses, or, if an illness is too far advanced, at least alleviate pain in a substantial way. The testimonials presented in this book have shown this clearly. Since the body is a conductor in general (unless the skin is very dry), I would like to take a moment to describe how electrons move in a conductor.

Let's take first the example of a 9-volt battery. Take a copper wire, fit a resistor on to it, and connect the ends to the positive and negative terminals of the battery. The current starts flowing from the positive terminal to the negative terminal of the battery. Positive charges are what make the copper material itself and so they cannot move. But the electrons move. They leave the negative terminal and flow to the positive terminal through the wire. Their motion is regulated by the resistor. Without it, all electrons in the battery would travel to the positive terminal at the same time, melting the copper wire. If you touched the wire, you would get burned. In this complex situation, the current is thought by many people to be the positive charges flowing from the positive terminal to the negative terminal. However, it is the electrons that are moving from the *negative* terminal to the *positive* terminal that produce the current. The misconception dates back to dear old Benjamin Franklin who, through his experiments with kites and not knowing the exact nature of electricity, thought that a positively charged electric "fluid" was flowing into the wire. We know now that electrons are always the flowing entities when there is a current in a conducting wire. The velocity of electrons moving into the wire is very slow. For a copper wire of radius 1 millimeter (mm) carrying a steady current of 10 amps, the drift velocity is only about 0.24 mm/sec—a quarter of a mm per second! And yet the current flows extremely fast.

To explain how it is possible that a slow electron flow can nevertheless produce a very fast current, I will use the example of a person who is grounded. In this case, the human body plays the role of the copper wire (and the resistor as well, because the body is not as good a conductor as copper). The negative terminal is the Earth. The positive terminal is represented by the EMFs or positively charged particles in the atmosphere. The protection against EMFs or positive charged particles offered by the Earth connection is established almost at the speed of light (186,000 miles/second). This means the electric current flowing through the body to cancel the effects of the EMFs or the positive particles is almost instantaneous. Knowing that even in such an excellent conductor as copper electrons move very slow, how can this be? An analogy may help our understanding. In Figure B-2, a straw is filled with small beads. The diameter of the straw accommodates the beads only in a line.

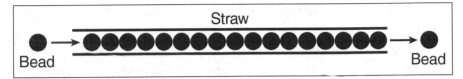

Figure B-2. The "straw-bead" effect. A bead introduced into the left end of the straw moves very little yet the bead at the far right end pops out almost instantly.

If you push the bead on the left side into the full straw, a bead pops out the other side almost instantaneously. The entering bead on the left has moved only a little (it is now the last bead inside the straw on the left side) and yet the *current* of beads has moved very fast. The last bead on the right side was pushed out almost instantaneously. Each bead inside the straw moved a distance of one bead diameter only and yet the *current* of beads (the propagation of the small movements of each bead) has moved through the straw almost instantaneously. All the beads inside the straw moved forward almost simultaneously. This is more or less how electrons move in a conductor. Electrons repel each other because they have the same negative electric charge. Because of this repelling effect between electrons, when an electron moves forward, it pushes forward all electrons ahead of it, just like the left bead pushed forward all the beads in the straw. This is what happens in a wire connected to both terminals of a battery. The slow movement of electrons in a wire also happens in the body and yet, at the same time, their slow movement collectively produces a fast current because of a "bead-straw" effect. The body is protected almost instantaneously by grounding because the fast current cancels out the effects of EMFs and/or the positive particles quickly. The electrons themselves take time to drift into the body.

The slow drift velocity of electrons helps explain a few observations in regard to Earthing.

1. It takes about twenty to thirty minutes for the healing response to start once a person is grounded. It may be, as explained in the section "Promoting the Body's Energy Fuel—ATP" in Chapter 11, that the metabolism utilizes electrons for proper function in bio-energy production and that it takes that much time for electrons to actually reach the area where metabolic activity is taking place. If conductive patches are placed

on the bottom of the feet, electrons start moving upward and sooner or later will push into the site where a specific problem exists. We assume the mitochondria around the problematic area will utilize the extra electrons in order to reinforce healing and repair activities. The process of infusing the mitochondria with additional electrons may take time. We do not know the exact mechanisms precisely involved but we know it takes between twenty and thirty minutes for the healing response to start when grounding is initiated.

2. When people stand or sit on the Earth, or are grounded via electrode patches placed on the soles of their feet, they often start feeling tingling and warmth rise in their body. The sensation starts in the feet, then progresses to the shins and calves, and after several minutes reaches the head.

3. Grounding speeds wound healing. Wounds heal faster than normal (ungrounded) when someone sleeps grounded, for instance on a grounded sheet, or applies a grounded electrode patch on the soles of the feet. The healing response is faster yet if the patches are placed near the wound. A dramatic example of that has been presented in Chapter 13 regarding a cyclist in the 2005 Tour de France who suffered severe lacerations to his upper right arm.

The same observation can be made for inflammation. Inflammation of the elbow, for example, will clear with the feet touching the ground. However, the inflammatory condition will be dissipated much faster if grounded electrode patches are placed next to the elbow. For the interested reader, more details on inflammation and how it is impacted by Earthing can be found in a 2007 article written by James Oschman in the *Journal of Alternative and Complementary Medicine* ("Can Electrons Act as Antioxidants? A Review and Commentary" 13: 955–967).

For additional information regarding the physics of grounding, please visit the Earthing Institute website at www.earthinginstitute.net.

Resources

The Earthing Institute (www.earthinginstitute.net)

The Institute website provides information for obtaining Earthing devices and tips on staying Earthed in any situation.

Readers are invited to visit this site—Earthing's official website—to learn about the newest developments and scientific studies regarding Earthing as they unfold.

The Institute plans also to provide certification of safety and effectiveness of various Earthing products supplied by manufacturers.

The Institute envisions offering online training of technicians in the theories and technology of Earthing and installation of Earthing devices. While such devices are simple for most anyone to install and utilize, issues related to inadequate electrical grounding systems in homes and offices are frequently encountered. The website will provide details on the programs, which will include training at basic, intermediate, and advanced levels.

Symptom Checklist and Progress Log

To assess how grounding may be helping you, list any common symptoms you have in the column on the left. In the second column, make a note of the severity of the problem. If the symptom is pain, for instance, rate the pain on a scale of 0 to 10. Then rate the condition or symptom one week and one month after grounding. You may also want to keep track of key medical tests the same way.

OBSERVATIONS			
CONDITION/ SYMPTOM	**PRE- GROUNDING**	**1 WEEK AFTER GROUNDING**	**1 MONTH AFTER GROUNDING**

APPENDIX E

Selected
Bibliography

Chapter 1

Franceschi C, Bonafe M, Valensin S, et al. "Inflamm-aging: an evolutionary perspective on immunosenescence." *Annals New York Academy of Sciences* 2006; 908: 244–254

Gorman C and Park A. "The fires within." *Time,* Feb 23, 2004; 38–46

Meggs W. *The Inflammation Cure.* New York: McGraw-Hill, 2004

Oschman JL. "Our place in Nature: reconnecting with the Earth for better sleep." *Journal of Alternative and Complementary Medicine* 2003; 10(5): 735–36

Suckling EE. *The Living Battery—An Introduction to Bioelectricity.* New York: Macmillan, 1964

Chapter 2

Bach JF. "Why is the incidence of autoimmune diseases increasing in the modern world?" *Endocrine Abstracts* 2008; 16(S3): 1

Bower B. "Slumber's unexplored landscape." *Science News Online* Sept 25, 1999

Gish OH. "The natural electric currents in the Earth. *Scientific Monthly* 1936; 43(1): 47–57

Max Planck Institutes. Research cited in *Energy Medicine: The Scientific Basis* by James L. Oschman (Churchill Livingstone, 2000): 101

Stein R. "Is modern life ravaging our immune systems?" *Washington Post* Mar 4, 2008

Tavera M. "The sacred mission"(translated by George Verdon) *ESD Journal* 2008; http://www.esdjournal.com/articles/sacredmission.htm

Williams ER and Heckman SJ. "The local diurnal variation of cloud electrification and the global diurnal variation of negative charge on the earth." *Journal of Geophysical Research* 1993; 98: 5221–5234

Chapter 4

Cho HJ, Lavretsky H, Olmstead R, et al. "Sleep disturbance and depression recurrence in community-dwelling older adults: a prospective study." *American Journal of Psychiatry* 2008; 165(12): 1543–1550

Ghaly M and Teplitz D. "The biologic effects of grounding the human body during sleep as measured by cortisol levels and subjective reporting of sleep, pain and stress." *Journal of Alternative and Complementary Medicine* 2004; 10(5): 767–776

Irwin MR, Wang M, Ribeiro D, et al. "Sleep loss activates cellular inflammatory signaling." *Biological Psychiatry* 2008; 64(6): 538–540

Ober AC. "Grounding the human body to earth reduces chronic inflammation and related chronic pain." *ESD Journal* Jul 2003; http://www.esdjournal.com/articles/cober/earth.htm

Ober AC. "Grounding the human body to neutralize bio-electrical stress from static electricity and EMFs." *ESD Journal* Jan 2000; http://www.esdjournal.com/articles/cober/ground.htm

Simpson N and Dinges DF. "Sleep and inflammation." *Nutrition Review* 2007; 65(12, part II): S244–52

Chapter 6

Amalu W. "A pilot study test of grounding the human body to reduce inflammation." Unpublished data

Omoigui S. "The origin of all pain is inflammation and the inflammatory response: a unifying law of pain." *Medical Hypotheses* 2007; 69: 70–82

Oschman JL. "Charge transfer in the living matrix." *Journal of Bodywork and Movement Therapies* 2009; 13: 215–28

Pischinger A. *Extracellular Matrix and Ground Regulation: Basis for a Holistic Biological Medicine.* Berkeley, CA: North Atlantic Books, 2007 (revised and updated English translation of *Das System der Grundregulation: Grundlagen für eine ganzheitsbiologische Theorie der Medizin,* originally published by K.F. Haug, Heidelberg, 1975)

Ridker PM et al. "Inflammation, aspirin, and the risk of cardiovascular-disease in apparently healthy men." *New England Journal of Medicine* 1997; 336(14): 973–79

Ridker PM et al. "C-reactive protein and other markers of inflammation in the prediction of cardiovascular disease in women." *New England Journal of Medicine* 2000; 342(12): 836–843

Salvioli S et al. "Inflamm-aging, cytokines and aging: state of the art, new hypotheses on the role of mitochondria and new perspectives from systems biology." *Current Pharmaceutical Design* 2006; 12(24): 3161–3171

Chapter 7

Applewhite R. "The effectiveness of a conductive patch and a conductive bed pad in reducing induced human body voltage via the application of earth ground." *European Biology and Bioelectromagnetics* 2005; 1: 23–40

Brown R, Chevalier G, Hill M. "Pilot study on the effect of grounding on delayed onset muscle soreness." *Journal of Alternative and Complementary Medicine* April 2010

Chevalier G, Mori K, Oschman, JL. "The effect of earthing (grounding) on human physiology." *European Biology and Bioelectromagnetics* January 31, 2006; 600–621

Chevalier G and Mori K. "The effect of earthing on human physiology (part II): electrodermal measurements." *Subtle Energy and Energy Medicine* 2007; 18(3): 11–34

Chevalier G. "Changes in pulse rate, respiratory rate, blood oxygenation, perfusion index, skin conductance and their variability induced during and after grounding human subjects for forty minutes." *Journal of Alternative and Complementary Medicine* January 2010

Feynman R, Leighton RB, and Sands M. *The Feynman Lectures on Physics* (vol II). Reading, MA: Addison-Wesley Publishing, 1964: Chapter 9

Jamiesona KS, ApSimona HM, Jamiesona SS, et al. "The effects of electric fields on charged molecules and particles in individual microenvironments." *Atmospheric Environment* 2007; 41: 5224–5235

Ober AC. "Grounding the human body to neutralize bio-electrical stress from static electricity and EMFs." *ESD Journal* 2004; http://www.esdjournal.com/articles/cober/ground.htm

Ober AC and Coghill RW. "Does grounding the human body to earth reduce chronic inflammation and related chronic pain?" Presentation at the European Bioelectromagnetics Association Annual Meeting, November 12, 2003, Budapest, Hungary

Oschman JL. "Can electrons act as antioxidants? a review and commentary." *Journal of Alternative and Complementary Medicine* 2007; 13(9): 955–967

Oschman JL. Perspective. "Assume a spherical cow: the role of free or mobile electrons in bodywork, energetic and movement therapies." *Journal of Bodywork and Movement Therapies* 2008; 12: 40–57

Oschman JL and Kessler WD. "Energy medicine and anti-aging: from fundamentals to new breakthroughs." *Anti-Aging Medical News* Winter 2008: 166–171

Chapter 8

Yang J. "No shoes? No problem." July 15, 2009; http:// www.theglobeandmail.com/ life/health/no-shoes-no-problem/article1219575/

Chapter 11

Chevalier G and Sinatra ST. "Emotional stress, heart rate variability, grounding, and improved autonomic tone." (In press)

Fontes A, Fernandes HP, et al. "Measuring electrical and mechanical properties of red blood cells with double optical tweezers." *Journal of Biomedical Optics* 2008; 13(1):014001

"Global high blood pressure situation growing dire, but doesn't have to be, new health report says." *Medical News Today* May 18, 2007; http://www.medicalnewstoday.com/ articles/71331.php

Shaper AG. "Cardiovascular disease in the tropics." *British Medical Journal* 1972; 4(5831): 32–35

Chapter 15

Puotinen CJ. "Earth energy." *Whole Dog Journal* January 2008: 17–21

Chapter 16

Beasley JD and Swift J. "The Kellogg Report: the impact of nutrition, environment & lifestyle on the health of Americans." Annandale-on-Hudson, NY: Bard College Center, Institute of Health Policy and Practice, 1989

Council of State Governments. "Costs of chronic diseases: what are states facing?" *Trends Alert* 2006

Appendix B

Fly Light Aviation Meteorology. "Atmospheric electricity"; www.auf.asn.au/ meteorology/ section11.html

McLafferty S and Wang F. "Rural reversal? Rural-urban disparities in late-stage cancer risk in Illinois." *Cancer* 2009; 115(12): 2755–2764

Wolinsky FD, Bentler SE, Cook EA, et al. "A 12-year prospective study of stroke risk in older Medicare beneficiaries." *BMC Geriatrics* May 9, 2009; 9: 17

Acknowledgments

To James Oschman, Ph.D., an extraordinary biophysicist, who has exhaustively researched the science related to the healing benefits of Earthing. He was the first to scientifically explain the transfer of free electrons from the Earth's pulsating surface into the electric matrix of the human body. His investigations, hypotheses, and published papers on the subject have given solid scientific basis to a paradigm-shifting health concept. Dr. Oschman is the director of Nature's Own Research Association in Dover, New Hampshire (www.energyresearch.bizland.com) and the author of *Energy Medicine: The Scientific Basis* (Churchill Livingstone, 2000) and *Energy Medicine in Therapeutics and Human Performance* (Butterworth-Heinemann, 2003). His work explores the existence of a high-speed communication system extending throughout the human body that responds to the energetic environment. Dr. Oschman holds a Ph.D. in biological sciences from the University of Pittsburgh. He is a member of the Scientific Advisory Board of the National Foundation for Alternative Medicine in Washington, D.C.

To Gaetan Chevalier, Ph.D., visiting researcher at the Developmental and Cell Biology Department, University of California at Irvine, and the keenest of biological investigators. His experiments and findings on the bioelectrical changes brought about by grounding have opened a new frontier of electrophysiological research examining the striking differences between grounded and nongrounded human beings. Dr. Chevalier holds a Ph.D. in engineering physics from the University of Montreal. He was formerly director of research at the California Institute for Human Science.

To Jeff Spencer, D.C., a master at improving the performance of elite athletes and making them more resistant to the ravages of fierce competition. His unique experience at the highest and most challenging level of sports dramatically demonstrates that optimum performance, whether on the playing field or in everyday activities, benefits immensely from Earthing. Jeff was named Sports Chiropractor of the Year in 2004 by the International Chiropractic Association.

To Jim Healy, a pre-eminent global figure in cutting-edge medical monitoring technology, for greatly appreciated guidance and support.

To Elizabeth Hughes, for sharing her very personal history of how Earthing relieved her from years of baffling ailments so common to many women, but especially for her tireless and dedicated assistance, in small ways and large, on behalf of Earthing research.

To Dick Brown, Ph.D., the internationally renowned exercise physiologist and trainer of elite athletes, whose research on delayed-onset muscle soreness documented the unique power of Earthing to reduce recovery time from injury.

To San Diego health researcher Dale Teplitz for being such an integral cog in Earthing's scientific detective work in the early days and beyond, and for sharing her dramatic story of healing, as well as her insights after leading many hundreds of individuals to the benefits of Earthing.

To old friends Corky and Kathleen Downing for support and enthusiasm over the years, and for helping show truckers and motorists how to bypass common driving tension and aches with a simple grounded seat pad.

To Sheila Curtiss and Bob Malone, for their stories and for being such staunch Earthing advocates for so long.

To Maurice Ghaly, M.D., the first doctor who took the time to consider the concept of Earthing and then report about its benefits in the medical literature.

To Russell Whitten, D.C., the first physician to apply Earthing in clinical practice and witness its great healing potential.

To Gabriel Cousens, M.D., David Gersten, M.D., Richard Delany, M.D., and Amanda Ward, N.D., for providing their experience with Earthing among patients.

To Bryan Moses, for introducing Earthing to the unique circle of people he helps to keep healthy.

To Bruce Beckert, a luminary in the fabric business, who has always been available, with patience, enthusiasm, and brilliance, to continually help refine the design and conductivity of Earthing devices.

To Nick and Carmen Warren, for sustained support and helping so much to locate and obtain the bits and pieces needed for ever-changing Earthing devices.

To John Gray, Ph.D., bestselling author of *Men Are From Mars, Women Are From Venus,* and healthy lifestyle guru David Wolfe, for sharing their Earthing stories.

To Arvord Belden, Roland Perez, Don Scott, Randy Gillett, Katherine Van Hatten, Jim Bellacera, Brad Graham, Ken Jones, Daryl James Jr., Lynne Corwin, Ron Petruccioni, Doree Lane, Anita Pointer, Howell Runion, Armida Champagne, John Steve Lopez, Steve Garner, Mike Miller, Roberta Mikkelsen, Jill Queen, Ted Barnett, Olivia Biera, Edie Miller, Mary Mason, Henry Falcon, Step Sinatra, Dean Levin, Stephanie and Chike Okeafor, Jim Schmedding, Cindy Walsh, Donna Tisdale, Jim Bagnola, Brianna Anderson-Gregg, and Scott Hyatt for taking the time to relate their Earthing stories.

To Dan and Tim Hall, and Dan Chittock, for valuable assistance in setting up contacts with Earthers.

To William Amalu, for validating the power of Earthing with thermography.

To Hugh Semple, for expertise in carrying out long-term laboratory studies.

To George Verdon, hale and hardy in his eighties, who has been spending countless barefoot hours in his garden over the last thirty years, for sharing with us his translation of the amazing insights of French agronomist Matteo Tavera.

To Mark Lindsay, for opening research doors.

To John Sullivan, for continuing support and videography.

To Jennifer Morris, for providing much appreciated administrative assistance.

To CJ Puotinen, a veteran pet writer and author, who has experienced how Earthing helps both four- and two-legged creatures.

To Norm Goldfind, a master of the publishing arts, for seeing the potential in our book.

To Cheryl Hirsch, for absolutely superb editing, and to Gary Rosenberg, for a beauty of a book.

To Mark Hinds and staff naturopath Anna Walden at the HealthWalk Integrative Wellness Center in Carlsbad, California, for providing zeta potential expertise and sophisticated instrumentation, plus much appreciated patience and assistance.

To Jack Weinberg for good friendship, a sharp eye, and for help ironing out assorted manuscript wrinkles, and to Fred Mendelsohn for also making valuable comments on the manuscript.

To Jack Scovil, the veteran New York literary agent and friend, for excellent advice as usual.

To Leya Booth, of Genius Office Services in Encino, California, for doing a spectacular and speedy job transcribing many interviews for a writer under the gun.

To Ruth Sharone, for lending a hand.

And to so many others, especially early on, who were willing to try the strange idea of a guy from the cable TV industry with no scientific or medical background who claimed that by standing barefoot on the Earth or sleeping on a bed pad or sheet connected to the Earth with a wire, you could actually sleep better, feel better, have less pain, and reduce multiple symptoms of illness.

Index

About the Authors

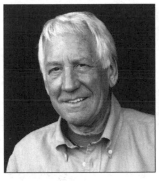

Clinton Ober started as a cable TV salesman in Billings, Montana, and rose to become a leader in the industry. In the early 1970s, he formed Telecrafter Corporation and built it into the largest provider of cable marketing and installation services in the United States. In the 1980s, he turned his attention to the fledgling computer industry. He partnered with McGraw-Hill to acquire live-feed distribution rights for computer use from news services around the world. Following a near fatal disease in 1993, he embarked on a personal journey looking for a higher purpose in life. During his travels, he discovered Earthing and has been resolutely focused ever since to promote the scientific exploration and practical applications for the concept.

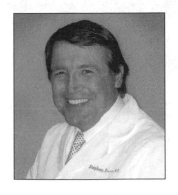

Stephen Sinatra, M.D., F.A.C.C., F.A.C.N., is a board-certified cardiologist and certified psychotherapist with more than thirty years of experience in helping patients prevent and reverse heart disease. He also is certified in anti-aging medicine and nutrition. Dr. Sinatra integrates conventional medical treatments for heart disease with complementary nutritional, anti-aging, and psychological therapies

259

that help heal the inflammation and plaque processes that cause heart attacks and stroke. He is a Fellow of the American College of Cardiology, an Assistant Clinical Professor of Medicine at the University of Connecticut School of Medicine, and a former chief of cardiology and medical education at Manchester (CT) Memorial Hospital. Dr. Sinatra has written numerous books, including *Reverse Heart Disease Now* (Wiley, 2008), *Lower Your Blood Pressure in Eight Weeks* (Ballantine Books, 2003), and *The Sinatra Solution: Metabolic Cardiology* (Basic Health, 2nd ed., 2008). He is also author of the popular nationally distributed newsletter *Heart, Health & Nutrition* and host of the heartmdinstitute.com website.

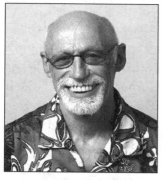

Martin Zucker has written extensively on natural healing, fitness, and alternative medicine for thirty years. He has co-authored or ghostwritten more than a dozen books, and written many video scripts for the National Safety Council. Among his latest books are *Move Yourself* and *Reverse Heart Disease Now* (both from John Wiley & Sons, 2008), *Natural Hormone Balance for Women* (Pocket Books, 2002), *The Miracle of MSM* (Berkley Trade, 1999), *Preventing Arthritis* (Berkley Trade, 2002), and *The Veterinarians' Guide to Natural Remedies for Dogs/Cats* (Three Rivers Press, 2000). Zucker has written hundreds of magazine articles on a wide variety of health topics and contributed to *Smithsonian, Readers Digest, Los Angeles Times, Cook's Magazine, Vegetarian Times, Muscle & Fitness, Men's Fitness,* and *The National Enquirer.* He is a former Associated Press foreign correspondent who worked in Europe and the Middle East.